Celiac
DISEASE
COOKBOOK

FOR THE NEWLY
DIAGNOSED

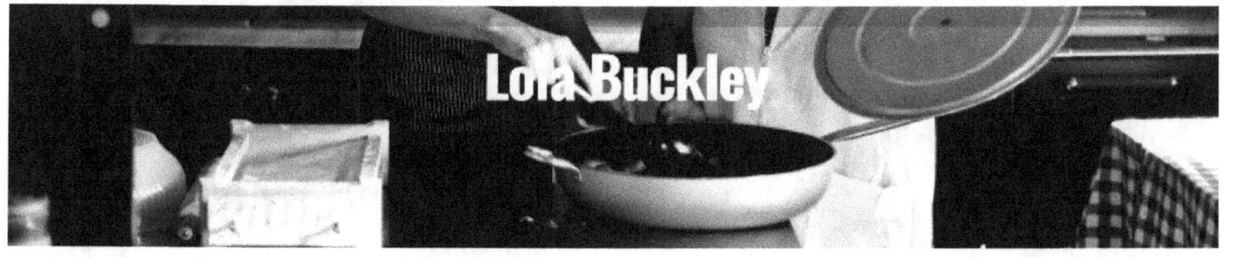

Table of Content

Introduction

The Discovery of Celiac Disease

The discovery of celiac disease is a fascinating, centuries-long adventure. Here are some important historical facts:

1. First Recorded Description Celiac disease was first described in ancient Greek medical texts by Aretaeus of Cappadocia around the 1st century AD. He documented a condition characterized by chronic diarrhea and malabsorption in children, which he attributed to a lack of assimilation of food.

2. Samuel Gee's contribution: In 1888, British physician Samuel Gee published one of the first modern descriptions of celiac disease. He identified the issue as a chronic digestive disorder and advised afflicted persons to eat rice, beef, mutton, and chicken broth, unwittingly recommending a gluten-free diet.

3. Willem Dicke's Research: During World War II, Dutch doctor Willem Dicke noticed that children with celiac disease showed improvement in symptoms during times of food scarcity, notably when wheat was unavailable owing to rationing. In 1950, he discovered a link between celiac disease and the ingestion of gluten-containing cereals.

4. Identifying Gluten as a Trigger: Dicke's study led to the discovery that gluten, a protein present in wheat, barley, and rye, is the cause of celiac disease. He anticipated that removing gluten from the diet would reduce symptoms and enhance the health of celiac patients.

5. Developing Diagnostic Tests: In the 1960s and 1970s, advances in medical technology resulted in the development of diagnostic procedures for celiac disease, such as serological testing to identify celiac-related antibodies in the blood and intestinal biopsies to assess small bowel damage.

6. Recognising Autoimmune Nature: Further study in the late twentieth century established that celiac disease is an autoimmune illness in which the body's immune system incorrectly assaults the lining of the small intestine in reaction to gluten consumption. This knowledge transformed the diagnosis and management of celiac disease.

7. Prevalence Study: In recent decades, epidemiological studies have given information on the global incidence of celiac disease. It is currently recognized as one of the most common chronic autoimmune illnesses, affecting around 1% of the world's population.

8. Advances in Treatment: Along with diagnostic breakthroughs, therapy options for celiac disease have changed. The cornerstone of therapy remains a gluten-free diet for life, although pharmacological breakthroughs, such as enzyme supplements and potential future medicines, give promise for better disease management.

The discovery of celiac disease has transformed our understanding of autoimmune disorders and revolutionized the approach to diagnosis and treatment, providing hope for better outcomes and quality of life for those affected by this condition.

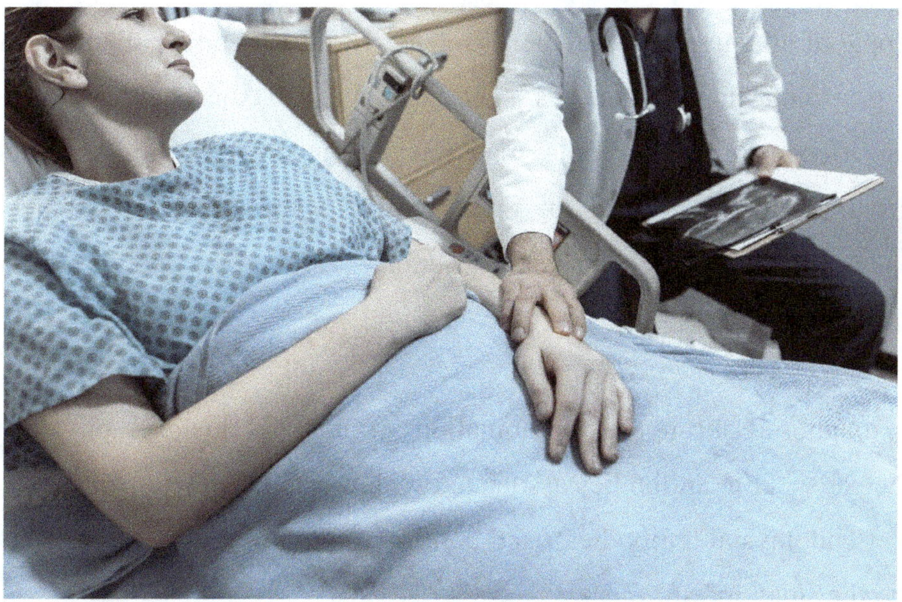

Chapter 1

Understanding Celiac Disease: Causes, Types, Symptoms, and Preventive Measures.

Celiac disease, also known as coeliac disease in some areas, is a chronic autoimmune condition defined by an inappropriate immune response to gluten, a protein present in wheat, barley, and rye. When people with celiac disease consume gluten, their immune system misidentifies it as a threat and initiates an immunological reaction that destroys the lining of the small intestine.

The small intestine is lined with tiny, finger-like extensions called villi, which are essential for absorbing nutrients from meals. In people with celiac disease, gluten triggers an immune response that causes inflammation and destruction to the villi, resulting in villous atrophy. As a result, the small intestine's ability to absorb nutrients decreases, which can cause a variety of symptoms and difficulties.

Celiac disease may affect people of all ages, from newborns to elderly adults, and it can show in a variety of ways. While gastrointestinal symptoms such as persistent diarrhea, stomach discomfort, and bloating are frequent, some people may develop unusual or non-specific symptoms that impact other organs and systems in their bodies. Symptoms may include dermatitis herpetiformis (an itchy, blistering skin rash), anemia, osteoporosis, neurological issues, infertility, and exhaustion.

Celiac disease is typically diagnosed through a combination of medical history, physical examination, blood tests to detect specific antibodies associated with the condition (such as anti-tissue transglutaminase or anti-endomysial antibodies), and confirmation via intestinal biopsy to assess the extent of damage to the small intestine.

Celiac illness can only be treated with a rigorous gluten-free diet for the rest of one's life. This includes avoiding any foods and goods containing wheat, barley, or rye, as well as cross-contamination with gluten-containing substances. Individuals suffering from celiac disease can successfully manage their symptoms, improve intestinal healing, and avoid long-term problems from the condition by following suitable dietary guidelines.

Individuals with celiac disease should collaborate closely with healthcare specialists such as gastroenterologists, dietitians, and nutritionists to ensure accurate diagnosis, treatment, and continuous management of the condition. Education on gluten-free living, label reading, and selecting safe food alternatives is critical for successfully managing celiac disease and enjoying a healthy, satisfying life.

Causes:

Celiac disease is an autoimmune illness affecting the small intestine that is caused by the consumption of gluten, a protein present in wheat, barley, and rye. The actual etiology of celiac disease is unknown, however, it is thought to be a mix of genetic, environmental, and immunological factors.

1. Genetic Factors: Celiac disease is mostly caused by a genetic predisposition. Individuals with certain genetic markers, particularly the human leukocyte antigen (HLA) genes HLA-DQ2 and HLA-DQ8, are more likely to acquire the disorder.
- Approximately 95% of people with celiac disease carry the HLA-DQ2 or HLA-DQ8 gene, however, possessing these genes does not ensure disease development.

2. Environmental Triggers: While genetics play an important role, environmental factors also influence the genesis of celiac disease. Consuming gluten-containing foods is a key environmental trigger. Gluten causes an immunological reaction in those with celiac disease, resulting in inflammation and damage to the lining of the small bowel. This damage inhibits nutrition absorption from diet and can result in a variety of symptoms.

3. Immune System Response: In celiac disease, the immune system incorrectly perceives gluten as a threat and responds against it. The immune response produces antibodies, including anti-tissue transglutaminase (tTG) and anti-endomysial antibodies (EMA), which target small intestinal tissues. Over time, this immune reaction causes inflammation and damage to the villi, which are tiny finger-like projections that border the small intestine and absorb nutrients from food.

4. Other Factors: - Celiac disease may be caused or aggravated by virus infections, childbirth, surgery, or extreme mental stress. These elements can alter the immune system's equilibrium and trigger symptoms in sensitive individuals. Furthermore, the timing of gluten intake in the diet, particularly during infancy, may influence the development of celiac disease. According to some research, introducing gluten into an infant's diet before four months or after seven months may raise the likelihood of having the illness.

While the precise interaction of genetic and environmental variables in celiac disease is complicated and poorly understood, it is known that both play important roles in its development. Understanding these factors is critical for early identification, diagnosis, and management of celiac disease, eventually increasing the quality of life for those who live with it.

Types:

Celiac disease is a complicated autoimmune ailment caused by an aberrant immune reaction to gluten, a protein present in wheat, barley, and rye. While the traditional form of celiac disease largely affects the small intestine, the disorder can emerge in a variety of ways, each with its own set of symptoms and features. Here are the primary kinds of celiac disease:

1. Classic Celiac Disease

Classic celiac disease is the normal manifestation of celiac disease, which includes gastrointestinal symptoms, malabsorption, and villous atrophy in the small intestine. This type of sickness is typically easier to identify because of the specific and strong symptoms it exhibits. Here is an explanation of the classic celiac disease.

1. Gastrointestinal symptoms: People with typical celiac disease frequently have a variety of gastrointestinal symptoms, such as persistent diarrhea, abdominal discomfort, bloating, gas, and nausea. These symptoms vary in intensity and length, but they are usually persistent and might worsen over time if not addressed.

2. Malabsorption: One of the characteristics of typical celiac disease is malabsorption, which develops when the small intestine's damaged lining is unable to effectively absorb nutrients from meals. This can cause deficits in critical vitamins, minerals, and other nutrients, leading to symptoms including weariness, weakness, and weight loss.

3. Villous atrophy: In typical celiac disease, gluten-induced inflammation and immune response cause destruction to the villi, which are tiny finger-like projections that border the small intestine and absorb nutrition. Over time, this damage causes villous atrophy, in which the villi flatten and lose their function.

4. The diagnosis is: Classic celiac disease is typically diagnosed through a combination of medical history, physical examination, blood tests to detect specific antibodies associated with the condition (such as anti-tissue transglutaminase or anti-endomysial antibodies), and confirmation via intestinal biopsy to assess the extent of small intestine damage.

5. Treatment: Classic celiac disease is treated mostly with a strict gluten-free diet for the rest of one's life. This includes avoiding all gluten-containing foods from the diet, such as wheat, barley, rye, and their derivatives. Individuals with typical celiac disease can successfully control their symptoms, improve intestinal healing, and avoid long-term problems from the condition by following suitable dietary guidelines.

6. Monitoring: Individuals with typical celiac disease may require regular monitoring by healthcare specialists, such as gastroenterologists and dietitians, to examine symptom management, nutritional status, and gluten-free diet compliance. Follow-up blood tests and intestinal biopsies may also be necessary to evaluate disease activity and ensure proper treatment.

Classic celiac disease is the classic presentation of the disorder, including gastrointestinal symptoms, malabsorption, and villous atrophy in the small intestine. Early identification, diagnosis, and adherence to a gluten-free diet are critical for controlling symptoms, facilitating healing, and increasing the quality of life in those with typical celiac disease.

2. Atypical Celiac Disease

Atypical celiac disease, also known as non-classic or silent celiac disease, is a form of illness in which patients suffer symptoms that are not predominantly gastrointestinal. Unlike traditional celiac disease, which is marked by severe gastrointestinal symptoms such as persistent diarrhea and abdominal discomfort, atypical celiac disease can cause a variety of symptoms affecting various organs and systems in the body. Here's an explanation for atypical celiac disease:

1. Non-gastrointestinal symptoms: Atypical celiac disease is frequently characterized by symptoms that affect organs and systems other than the gastrointestinal tract. Symptoms may include unexplained iron deficiency anemia, osteoporosis, dermatitis herpetiformis (a skin rash with itchy, blistering blisters), neuropathy (tingling, numbness, or pain in the hands and feet), weariness, joint discomfort, and infertility.

2. Variability in symptoms: The symptoms of atypical celiac disease vary greatly across individuals and may overlap with other medical disorders, making diagnosis difficult. Some people may have a variety of symptoms affecting multiple organs and systems of the body, whereas others may only have one or two uncommon symptoms.

3. Delayed Diagnosis: Because of the lack of conventional gastrointestinal symptoms, atypical celiac disease is frequently underdiagnosed or misdiagnosed, resulting in delayed diagnosis and treatment. Individuals with atypical celiac disease may require extensive testing and examination before getting a clear diagnosis, which can prolong symptoms and lower quality of life.

4. The diagnosis is: Atypical celiac disease is typically diagnosed through a combination of medical history, physical examination, blood tests to detect specific antibodies associated with the condition (such as anti-tissue transglutaminase or anti-endomysial antibodies), and

confirmation via intestinal biopsy to assess the extent of small intestine damage. Additional tests may be required to determine symptoms impacting different organs and systems in the body.

5. Treatment: Atypical celiac disease, like classic celiac disease, is treated primarily by adhering to a gluten-free diet for the rest of one's life. Eliminating gluten from the diet can help reduce symptoms, improve intestinal healing, and avoid long-term problems of the illness. Individuals with atypical celiac disease may benefit from nutritional supplements to correct any deficits caused by malabsorption.

6. Management of Associated Conditions: Individuals with atypical celiac disease may need to treat other problems such as iron deficiency anemia, osteoporosis, dermatitis herpetiformis, and neuropathy in addition to maintaining a gluten-free diet. This might include medical interventions, nutritional adjustments, and lifestyle changes to improve general health and well-being.

Atypical celiac disease is a distinct form of the illness marked by symptoms that extend beyond the gastrointestinal system. Recognizing unusual symptoms and diagnosing them early is critical for successful care and better results for people with this kind of celiac disease.

3. Latent Celiac Disease

Latent celiac disease occurs when a person has a hereditary susceptibility to celiac disease and tests positive for celiac-related antibodies but does not have any symptoms or evidence of intestinal damage. Despite the lack of symptoms, people with latent celiac disease are at risk of acquiring active celiac disease later in life, especially if they continue to eat gluten-containing foods. This is an explanation of latent celiac disease.

Genetic Predisposition: Like classic and atypical celiac disease, latent celiac disease is linked to various genetic markers, most notably the HLA-DQ2 and HLA-DQ8 genes. Individuals with these genetic markers are more likely to acquire celiac disease than the general population, although not all of them will.

Positive Celiac-Related Antibodies: Individuals with latent celiac disease may be positive for celiac-related antibodies, such as anti-tissue transglutaminase (tTG) or anti-endomysial antibodies (EMA), suggesting an immunological response to gluten. They do not currently have celiac disease symptoms, and a biopsy may not reveal indications of intestinal damage.

No Symptoms: Unlike classic and atypical celiac disease, people with latent celiac disease do not have gastrointestinal symptoms or other common symptoms linked with the disorder. This lack of symptoms might make identification difficult since people may not seek medical treatment or tests for celiac disease.

Increased Risk of Active Disease: Individuals with latent celiac disease may not have symptoms or intestinal damage right now, but they are nonetheless at risk of developing active celiac disease later in life. Continued gluten intake can cause symptoms to appear and eventually lead to intestinal damage, especially if left untreated.

Monitoring and follow-up: Individuals with latent celiac disease may require ongoing monitoring and follow-up with healthcare specialists, such as gastroenterologists and dietitians, to determine their risk of acquiring active illness. Periodic blood tests to monitor celiac-related antibodies, as well as intestinal biopsies, may be indicated to identify changes in disease activity.

Considerations for a Gluten-Free Diet: Individuals with latent celiac disease may not need to follow a gluten-free diet right now, but they may choose to do so as a preventative step to lower their chance of acquiring active illness. A gluten-free diet may reduce inflammation and immunological reactions, perhaps delaying or avoiding the onset of symptoms and intestinal damage.

Latent celiac disease is a distinct clinical entity defined by a hereditary propensity to celiac disease but no current symptoms or intestinal damage. Early identification, frequent monitoring, and lifestyle changes, such as adopting a gluten-free diet, can help minimize the chance of developing active celiac disease and improve long-term results for those with the illness.

Potential celiac disease (PCD) is a condition in which people test positive for celiac-related antibodies and/or exhibit modest abnormalities in the small intestine but may not match the criteria for a confirmed diagnosis of celiac disease. This group covers those who have early or minor indicators of the disorder, as well as those who do not have symptoms despite evidence of an immunological response to gluten. Here's an explanation of possible celiac disease.

Positive Celiac-Related Antibodies: Individuals with suspected celiac disease usually test positive for celiac-related antibodies, such as anti-tissue transglutaminase (tTG) or anti-endomysial antibodies (EMA), which indicate an immunological response to gluten. These antibodies can be discovered by blood tests or serological testing.

Mild Abnormalities of the Small Intestine In addition to positive celiac-related antibodies, patients with probable celiac disease may have modest abnormalities in the small intestine on biopsy, such as increased intraepithelial lymphocytes (IELs) or moderate villous blunting. However, these alterations may not be sufficient for a definite diagnosis of celiac disease, which often needs more severe damage to the intestinal lining.

No Symptoms: Unlike classic or atypical celiac disease, people with possible celiac disease may not have gastrointestinal symptoms or other recognized signs of the disorder. This lack of symptoms might make identification difficult, since people may not seek medical care or tests for celiac disease until later in life.

 Increased Risk of Active Disease: Individuals with probable celiac disease are thought to have a higher chance of having active celiac disease later in life, particularly if they continue to consume gluten-containing foods. Continued gluten intake can precipitate the onset of symptoms and cause more severe intestinal damage over time.

Monitoring and follow-up: Individuals with suspected celiac disease may need regular monitoring and follow-up with healthcare specialists, such as gastroenterologists and dietitians, to determine their risk of developing active illness. Periodic blood tests to monitor celiac-related antibodies, as well as intestinal biopsies, may be indicated to identify changes in disease activity.

Considering a Gluten-Free Diet: Individuals with probable celiac disease may not need to follow a gluten-free diet right now, but they may choose to do so as a preventative step to lower their chance of acquiring active illness. A gluten-free diet may reduce inflammation and immunological reactions, perhaps delaying or avoiding the onset of symptoms and intestinal damage.

Potential celiac disease is a distinct clinical entity defined by positive celiac-related antibodies and/or modest abnormalities in the small intestine in the absence of current symptoms or a confirmed diagnosis of celiac disease. Early identification, frequent monitoring, and lifestyle changes, such as adopting a gluten-free diet, can help minimize the chance of developing active celiac disease and improve long-term results for those with the illness.

5. Refractory Celiac Disease

Refractory celiac disease (RCD) is an uncommon and significant complication of celiac disease that is distinguished by chronic or recurring symptoms and villous atrophy in the small intestine despite a rigorous gluten-free diet. Unlike normal celiac disease, which usually responds favorably to dietary adjustments, refractory celiac disease may not improve with gluten avoidance and may require further medical intervention. This is an explanation of refractory celiac disease.

Persistent Symptoms: Despite adhering to a rigorous gluten-free diet, people with refractory celiac disease continue to suffer symptoms such as diarrhea, stomach discomfort, bloating, exhaustion, and loss of weight. These symptoms can be severe and debilitating, reducing the quality of life and general well-being.

Villous Atrophy: Refractory celiac disease is distinguished by chronic or recurrent villous atrophy in the small intestine, as shown by biopsy. This implies persistent damage to the intestinal lining, which inhibits nutritional absorption and can result in malnutrition and other consequences.

Two subtypes: Refractory celiac disease is classified into two subgroups depending on the presence of aberrant intraepithelial lymphocytes (IELs) in the small intestine. Type I RCD is distinguished by normal or slightly elevated IELs, but Type II RCD is distinguished by clonal growth of aberrant IELs, comparable to lymphoma.

The diagnosis is: Refractory celiac disease is often diagnosed by clinical assessment, serological testing, endoscopic biopsy, and the elimination of other probable sources of symptoms. Blood tests may demonstrate high levels of celiac-related antibodies, and a biopsy may reveal ongoing villous atrophy despite a gluten-free diet.

Treatment: Treatment for refractory celiac disease is determined by its subtype and severity. In certain circumstances, further dietary changes, such as avoiding lactose or other food triggers, may be suggested. Immunomodulatory medicines, such as corticosteroids, immunosuppressants, or biologic therapies, may be used to suppress the immune response and reduce intestinal inflammation. In extreme situations, stem cell transplantation may be used as a last option.

Monitoring and follow-up: Individuals with refractory celiac disease require ongoing monitoring and follow-up with healthcare specialists, such as gastroenterologists and dietitians, to examine symptom management, nutritional status, and therapy response. Periodic blood tests and intestinal biopsies may be required to evaluate disease activity and alter therapy as necessary.

Complications: Untreated or poorly handled refractory celiac disease can result in major problems such as malnutrition, osteoporosis, immunological diseases, and an increased risk of intestinal cancer. Early diagnosis and care are critical for reducing complications and improving long-term results.

Refractory celiac disease is a difficult and complex disorder that needs specialist medical treatment and collaborative management. Individuals with refractory celiac disease can improve their quality of life by receiving correct diagnosis and treatment.

Understanding the many types of celiac disease is critical for proper diagnosis, effective treatment, and better results for those living with the condition. Early identification and care can help celiac patients avoid problems and improve their quality of life.

Symptoms:

The illness can generate a variety of symptoms that impact many bodily systems. Individuals with celiac disease might have a wide range of symptoms. Here are the most prevalent symptoms connected with the condition:

1. Gastrointestinal symptoms:
Symptoms may include chronic diarrhea or constipation.
- Abdominal ache and cramps.
- Bloating and Gas
- Nausea, vomiting.
- Indigestion.
- Bad-smelling or greasy feces (steatorrhea).
- Weight loss or inability to thrive (particularly in youngsters).

2. Malabsorption symptoms:
- Fatigue and weakness.
- Anemia (iron, B12, or folate deficiency)
- Osteoporosis or osteopenia (weak and brittle bones).
Symptoms may include muscle cramping and joint discomfort, as well as dental enamel flaws including discoloration or pitting.
- Easy bruising and sluggish wound healing.

3. Dermatologic Symptoms:
- Dermatitis herpetiformis (an itchy, blistering skin rash, usually on the elbows, knees, buttocks, or scalp).
- Eczema or psoriasis-like skin lesions.
- Dry and flaky skin.

- Mouth ulcers and canker sores

4. Neurological symptoms:

- Peripheral neuropathy (tingling, numbness, or pain in your hands and feet)

- Headaches and migraines.

- Cognitive impairment (brain fog, trouble focusing)

5. Reproductive symptoms:

- Adolescent delayed puberty or menstruation. - Infertility or repeated miscarriages.

- Erectile dysfunction or impotence in men.

6. Behavioral and Psychological Symptoms:

- Anxiety and Depression

Symptoms may include irritability, mood changes, and difficulty paying attention.

- Behavioral issues among youngsters

7. Other Symptoms:

- Fibromyalgia-like symptoms or chronic fatigue syndrome.

- Short stature or failure to flourish in children - Autoimmune illnesses (e.g., type 1 diabetes, autoimmune thyroid disease, or autoimmune hepatitis).

- Liver problems (increased liver enzymes)

It is crucial to note that not everyone with celiac disease has gastrointestinal symptoms. Some people may present with unusual or nonspecific symptoms affecting various organs and systems of the body, making diagnosis difficult. Furthermore, the severity and length of symptoms can vary greatly between individuals, and others may have moderate or intermittent symptoms.

Preventative Measures:

Currently, there is no treatment for Celiac disease, although it may be properly controlled with a strict gluten-free diet. The main objective of treatment is to remove gluten from the diet to avoid future damage to the small intestine and relieve symptoms. Here are some preventative measures and care options for people with celiac disease.

1. Adopting a Gluten-Free Diet: Managing Celiac illness requires avoiding all gluten-containing foods. This comprises foods made from wheat, barley, rye, and their derivatives. A gluten-free diet requires careful reading of product labels and awareness of hidden gluten sources.

2. Seeking Nutritional Guidance: Because Celiac disease can cause nutritional malabsorption, consulting with a licensed dietitian or nutritionist can assist ensure that people with Celiac disease get enough nutrition and manage any nutrient deficits.

3. Preventing Cross-Contamination: Individuals with Celiac disease must avoid cross-contamination since even trace quantities of gluten can cause symptoms. This includes utilizing separate cooking tools, cutting boards, and kitchen equipment for gluten-free items, as well as avoiding shared cooking surfaces in restaurants and food places.

4. Educate Others: Individuals with Celiac disease must educate their family, friends, and food service providers about the necessity of avoiding gluten and preventing cross-contamination. Clear communication and understanding can assist in establishing a friendly atmosphere for those with Celiac disease.

5. Regular Monitoring: Regular follow-up with healthcare practitioners is critical for tracking the progression of Celiac disease and identifying any problems or nutrient shortages. This may include blood testing to detect Celiac disease-related antibodies and periodic intestinal biopsies to assess the level of intestinal damage.

Individuals suffering from Celiac disease can successfully manage their illness, reduce symptoms, and enhance their overall quality of life by using these preventive measures and treatment tactics. Furthermore, continuing research into the underlying processes of Celiac disease and prospective therapeutic options provides promise for improved management and outcomes for people suffering from this chronic autoimmune ailment.

Advantages of Following a Celiac Disease Diet for Beginners

For those new to celiac disease, following a rigorous gluten-free diet is not only crucial for controlling the condition, but it also provides several health advantages. Individuals with celiac disease who eliminate gluten-containing foods from their diet can experience symptom relief, promote gut healing, prevent long-term complications, improve nutritional status, boost energy levels, support weight management, improve quality of life, and avoid accidental gluten exposure. Let's go further into each of these key advantages:

1. Relief from Symptoms:

Celiac disease causes a variety of symptoms, such as gastrointestinal discomfort, weariness, joint pain, and skin rashes. Beginners can find relief from these symptoms by following a gluten-free diet, which reduces inflammation in the small intestine and allows the body to recuperate. Symptoms such as diarrhea, bloating, stomach discomfort, and nausea are frequently relieved, resulting in increased comfort and well-being.

2. Supports Gut Healing:

The defining feature of celiac disease is damage to the small intestinal lining, which hinders nutritional absorption and can lead to problems if not addressed. Eliminating gluten from the diet helps the gut repair over time, regaining structure and function. As the intestine heals, people enjoy greater nutritional absorption, digestion, and inflammation reduction, which promotes overall gut health.

3. Prevents Long-Term Complications:

Untreated or poorly managed celiac disease can result in major long-term consequences such as malnutrition, osteoporosis, infertility, neurological issues, and certain malignancies. Beginners who follow a gluten-free diet can dramatically lower their chances of these issues while also maintaining superior overall health over time.

4. Boosts Nutritional Status:

Celiac disease can cause nutritional malabsorption, resulting in vitamin and mineral deficits. A gluten-free diet ensures that people with celiac disease consume a wide range of nutrient-dense, naturally gluten-free foods, such as fruits, vegetables, lean proteins, and gluten-free cereals. This promotes higher nutritional status, corrects any inadequacies, and improves general health and well-being.

5. Increases Energy Levels:

Many people with untreated celiac disease feel exhausted and have low energy levels as a result of malnutrition, inflammation, and the immune system's reaction. Beginners who follow a gluten-free diet and provide their bodies with the nutrients they require might feel enhanced energy, stamina, and general vitality, allowing them to participate in daily activities with greater ease and enjoyment.

6. Helps Weight Management:

Some people with celiac disease may lose or gain weight due to malabsorption, changes in appetite, or other causes. A gluten-free diet can help with weight management by encouraging good eating habits, appropriate nutrient absorption, and a balanced calorie intake. Beginners may reach and maintain a healthy weight by eating full, nutrient-dense meals and avoiding processed gluten-free goods that are heavy in sugar and bad fats.

7. Enhances Quality of Life:

Living with celiac disease can be difficult, but adopting a gluten-free diet can greatly improve the quality of life for both newcomers and those managing the condition. A gluten-free diet helps people to live more active, comfortable, and happy lives by lowering symptoms, eliminating complications, and increasing general health and well-being, free of the constraints and discomforts associated with untreated celiac disease.

8. Prevents Accidental Gluten Exposure.

Individuals with celiac disease must strictly adhere to a gluten-free diet to avoid accidental gluten consumption, which can induce symptoms and intestinal damage. To reduce the danger of gluten contamination, beginners should be cautious about their food selections, read labels carefully, and use safe food preparation practices. Individuals who take proactive steps to limit gluten exposure can retain the integrity of their diet and improve their health results.

Following a celiac disease diet provides numerous benefits for beginners, including symptom relief, gut healing, prevention of long-term complications, improved nutritional status, increased energy levels, weight management support, improved quality of life, and prevention of accidental gluten ingestion. Individuals with celiac disease may regain control of their health and well-being by adopting a gluten-free lifestyle and making informed dietary choices, resulting in a happier, healthier, and more satisfying life.

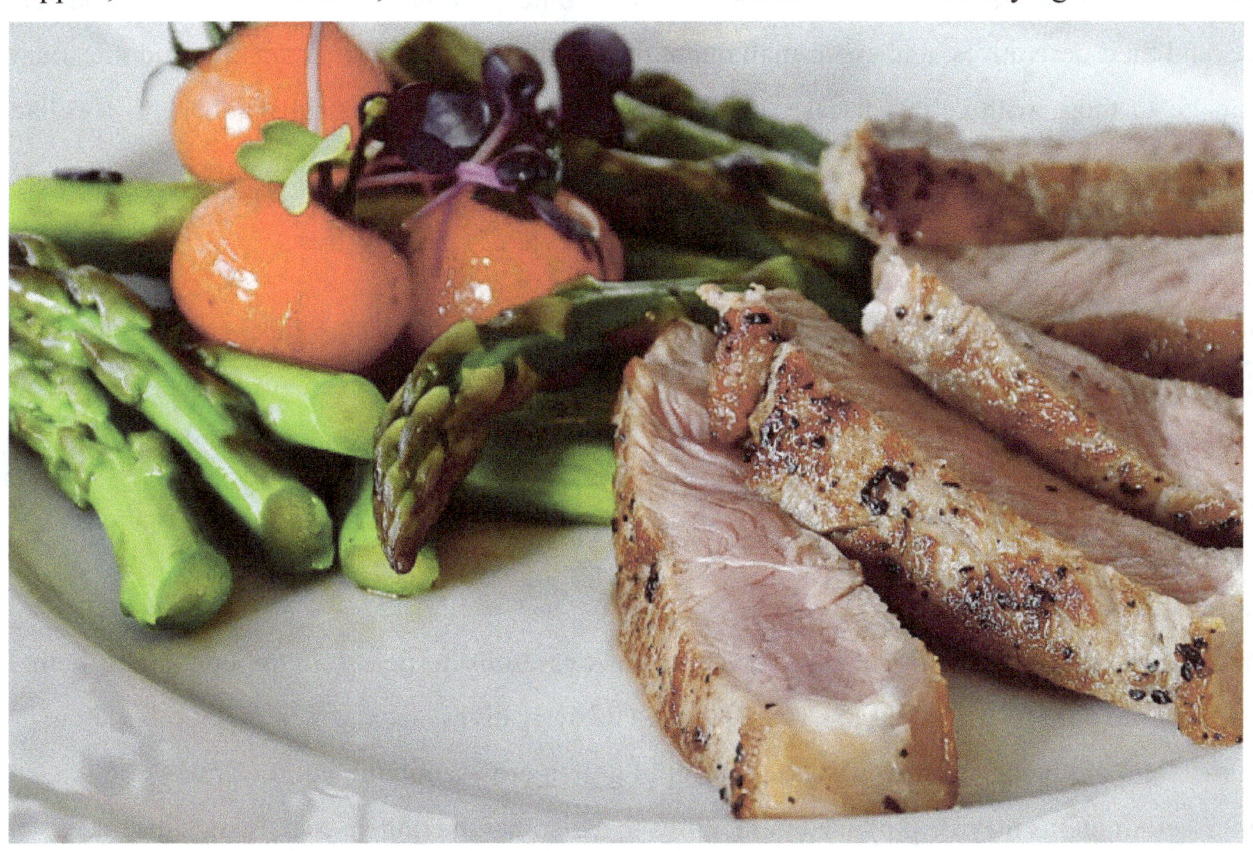

Chapter 2

Following Celiac Disease diet.

A celiac disease diet demands a rigorous commitment to a gluten-free lifestyle, which includes removing all gluten-containing foods from the diet. Gluten is a protein present in wheat, barley, rye, and their derivatives, and even small quantities of gluten can induce symptoms and intestinal damage in those with celiac disease. Here's how novices may successfully adhere to a celiac disease diet:

1. Educate Yourself:

Begin by learning more about celiac illness, gluten-containing foods, and gluten-free alternatives. Learn to identify typical sources of gluten in foods and beverages, as well as hidden sources of gluten in processed and packaged goods. Understanding the fundamentals of a gluten-free diet is critical for successfully managing celiac disease.

2. Read the Labels Carefully:

When supermarket shopping, always read the labels carefully to detect gluten-containing items. Look for the phrases wheat, barley, rye, malt, and its derivatives, such as wheat flour, barley malt extract, and rye bread crumbs. Also, be careful of gluten cross-contamination warnings on labels, since certain items may be produced in facilities that also handle gluten-containing substances.

3. Eat naturally gluten-free foods such as fruits, vegetables, lean proteins, dairy products, grains, legumes, nuts, and seeds. These foods include necessary nutrients and can serve as the foundation for a gluten-free diet that is both balanced and healthy. Experiment with different recipes and cooking methods to add a diversity of flavors and textures to your dishes.

4. Select Certified Gluten-Free Products:

Choose packaged and processed foods that have been gluten-free and verified by reliable organizations. Look for gluten-free certification marks or seals on food packaging to confirm that the product has been tested and satisfies rigorous gluten-free requirements. Certified gluten-free items ensure that they are safe for celiac disease patients to eat.

5. Avoid cross-contamination:

Take steps to avoid cross-contamination in the kitchen and while dining out. To minimize cross-contamination, use gluten-free cooking utensils, cutting boards, and kitchen equipment. Be cautious of shared cooking surfaces, condiment containers, and cooking oils that may be contaminated with gluten. When dining out, convey your dietary requirements to the restaurant personnel and inquire about gluten-free alternatives and food preparation methods.

6. Plan:

Plan your meals and snacks ahead of time to ensure that gluten-free choices are accessible when you're hungry. Fill your cupboard, refrigerator, and freezer with gluten-free essentials and supplies for quick and simple meal preparation. Consider bulk cooking and meal preparation to save time and make gluten-free eating easier during hectic days.

7. Seek Help and Resources:

Contact support groups, internet forums, and celiac disease organizations for advice, encouragement, and resources. Connect with people who eat gluten-free and exchange ideas, recipes, and experiences. Additionally, contact a licensed dietitian or nutritionist who specializes in celiac disease for specific nutritional advice and assistance.

8. Stay Positive and Persistent.

Adjusting to a gluten-free lifestyle can be difficult, especially at first, but remaining optimistic and persistent is essential for success. Concentrate on the advantages of adopting a celiac disease diet, such as symptom reduction, better health, and a higher quality of life. Celebrate minor triumphs along the road, and remember that with patience and practice, gluten-free eating will become second nature.

By following these steps and making educated dietary decisions, beginners may successfully navigate a celiac disease diet, manage their illness, and live a healthy and satisfying gluten-free lifestyle.

Shopping Ingredients

Shopping for a celiac disease diet entails paying close attention to ingredient labels and choosing goods that are naturally gluten-free or certified gluten-free. Here are 20 healthy shopping ingredients and meal lists appropriate for people with celiac disease:

1. Gluten-Free Grains:

Select gluten-free grains such as brown rice, quinoa, millet, amaranth, buckwheat, and certified gluten-free oats. These grains are flexible and healthful and may serve as the foundation for a variety of foods such as grain bowls, salads, and side dishes.

2. Fresh fruit and vegetables:

Stock up on fresh fruits and vegetables such as leafy greens, berries, citrus fruits, apples, bananas, carrots, broccoli, and bell peppers. These nutrient-dense meals provide critical vitamins, minerals, antioxidants, and fiber, which promote general health and well-being.

3. Lean protein:

Lean protein sources include fowl (chicken, turkey), fish (salmon, trout, and tuna), eggs, tofu, tempeh, legumes (beans and lentils), and nuts. These protein-rich meals are necessary for muscle repair, immunological function, and general health.

4. Dairy Alternatives:

Choose lactose-free dairy products or dairy substitutes fortified with calcium and vitamin D, such as lactose-free milk, yogurt, and cheese, as well as fortified plant-based milk alternatives like almond milk, soy milk, or coconut milk.

5. Gluten-Free Pasta and Grains:

Look for gluten-free pasta made with rice, maize, quinoa, or legumes, as well as gluten-free grains such as rice noodles, quinoa flakes, polenta, and cornmeal. These gluten-free options have the same texture and taste as regular pasta and grains.

6. Cans and dried beans/legumes:

Stock up on canned and dried beans and legumes, including chickpeas, black beans, kidney beans, lentils, and split peas. These pantry staples include protein, fiber, and important nutrients and may be used in soups, stews, salads, and side dishes.

7. Gluten-free Flour and Baking Ingredients:

Gluten-free flours and baking ingredients are ideal for making gluten-free baked products and sweets. Look for ingredients like almond flour, coconut flour, rice flour, tapioca flour, potato starch, and xanthan gum to use in bread, muffins, pancakes, and sweets.

8. Nut & Seed Butters:

Choose nut and seed butter produced with almonds, cashews, peanuts, sunflower, or pumpkin seeds. These spreads taste great on gluten-free bread, rice cakes, or fruit slices and include healthy fats, protein, and important elements.

9. Gluten-Free Snacks:

Search for gluten-free snacks and convenience foods such as rice cakes, popcorn, gluten-free crackers, rice crisps, veggie chips, nuts, seeds, and dried fruit. These snacks are ideal for on-the-go snacking and will satisfy cravings without jeopardizing your gluten-free diet.

10. Herbs, spices, and seasonings:

Stock your pantry with a variety of herbs, spices, and seasonings to enhance the flavor and richness of your gluten-free recipes. To improve the flavor of your food, consider using basil, oregano, thyme, rosemary, garlic powder, onion powder, paprika, turmeric, and cinnamon.

11. Gluten-free condiments & sauces:

Check the labels for gluten-free condiments and sauces including ketchup, mustard, mayonnaise, salsa, marinara sauce, barbecue sauce, tamari (gluten-free soy sauce), and salad dressings. Many manufacturers provide gluten-free versions of these goods to help people with celiac disease.

12. Gluten-Free Cereals and Granola:

Look for gluten-free cereals and granola prepared using gluten-free grains such as rice, maize, quinoa, and certified gluten-free oats. These breakfast options are a quick and healthy way to start the day and may be served with milk or dairy-free alternatives.

13. Gluten-Free Baking Mixes:

Discover gluten-free baking mixes for quick and simple baking tasks, such as gluten-free pancake mix, muffin mix, cake mix, and cookie mix. These pre-made mixes make gluten-free baking easier and more consistent, eliminating the need to measure individual ingredients.

14. Gluten-Free Pizza Crusts and Bread:

Find gluten-free pizza crusts and bread alternatives to make delicious gluten-free meals. Look for frozen or fresh gluten-free pizza crusts made with cauliflower, rice, or gluten-free flour, as well as gluten-free bread made with rice, quinoa, or almond flour.

15. Gluten-Free Ready Meals:

Keep an eye out for gluten-free ready dinners and entrees in the grocery store's freezer or refrigerator department. These practical solutions allow you to enjoy gluten-free meals at home without losing taste or quality.

16. Gluten-Free Desserts and Treats:

Enjoy gluten-free pastries and delights such as cookies, brownies, cakes, and ice cream. Many businesses provide gluten-free versions of popular sweets, allowing celiac patients to fulfill their sweet desires without jeopardizing their diet.

17. Gluten-Free Drinks:

Drink gluten-free water, herbal tea, coffee, 100% fruit juice, vegetable juice, coconut water, and gluten-free alcoholic beverages including wine, cider, and gluten-free beer. These solutions offer hydration and refreshment without gluten.

18. Gluten-free Frozen Fruits & Vegetables:
Stock your freezer with gluten-free frozen fruits and veggies for quick and easy meal prep. Frozen berries, spinach, broccoli, peas, and maize maintain their nutritional content and are ideal for smoothies, stir-fries, and side dishes.

19. gluten-free soups and broths:
Look for gluten-free soups and broths prepared with vegetables, meat, beans, and gluten-free grains. These ready-to-eat choices give warmth and comfort on chilly days and may be eaten on their own or with gluten-free bread or crackers.

20. Gluten-free, dairy-free alternatives:
Consider dairy-free alternatives to regular dairy products for celiac patients who also have lactose intolerance or dairy allergies. Choose from almond milk, soy milk, coconut milk, dairy-free yogurt, and cheese made from nuts or seeds.

Individuals suffering from celiac disease can enjoy a broad and nutritious gluten-free eating plan that benefits their health and well-being by including these healthy shopping ingredients and meal lists in their diet. Beginners may make informed choices while shopping for fresh fruit, pantry staples, or gluten-free convenience items to suit their dietary needs while still enjoying tasty gluten-free meals and snacks.

Complications of Celiac Disease, if the right diet isn't adopted

Celiac disease is a chronic autoimmune ailment marked by a sensitivity to gluten, a protein present in wheat, barley, rye, and their derivatives. When people with celiac disease ingest gluten-containing foods, their immune system produces an aberrant reaction that destroys the lining of the small intestine, resulting in inflammation and decreased nutritional absorption. While adhering to a rigorous gluten-free diet is essential for controlling celiac disease, failing to do so can result in a variety of short- and long-term consequences. Here are some of the issues that may occur if the proper diet is not followed:

1. Persistent Gastrointestinal Symptoms:

Individuals with celiac disease who do not follow a rigorous gluten-free diet are more prone to suffer from chronic gastrointestinal symptoms such as diarrhea, stomach discomfort, bloating, and nausea. These symptoms can have a major influence on quality of life, interfering with everyday tasks and social interactions.

2. Malnutrition and nutrient deficiencies:

Damage to the small intestine's lining limits nutritional absorption, resulting in malnutrition and shortages of vitamins, minerals, and other vital elements. Individuals with celiac disease who do not receive correct treatment may develop iron, calcium, vitamin D, vitamin B12, folate, and other nutritional deficiencies, which can lead to anemia, osteoporosis, lethargy, weakness, and other health issues.

3. Weight loss or gain:

Unintentional weight loss or gain can occur in people with untreated or poorly controlled celiac disease. Malabsorption of nutrients, variations in appetite, and metabolic abnormalities can all contribute to swings in body weight, which can have a severe impact on general health and well-being.

4. Untreated celiac disease can cause chronic inflammation and immunological dysregulation, leading to increased vulnerability to infections and autoimmune illnesses. Celiac disease patients may face more frequent infections, longer recovery periods, and a higher risk of secondary autoimmune disorders such as type 1 diabetes, autoimmune thyroiditis, and autoimmune liver disease.

5. Osteoporosis and Bone Disorders:

Untreated celiac disease can cause osteoporosis, which is characterized by weak and brittle bones, as well as other bone problems such as osteopenia and osteomalacia. Malabsorption of calcium and vitamin D, along with chronic inflammation, can lead to bone loss and raise the risk of fractures, especially in older persons.

6. Neurological and Psychiatric Disorders:
Celiac disease is associated with neurological and psychological diseases such as peripheral neuropathy, migraine headaches, depression, anxiety, and cognitive impairment. Untreated celiac disease can worsen these disorders, resulting in persistent neurological symptoms, cognitive impairment, and poor mental health outcomes.

7. Infertility and Reproductive Issues:
Celiac illness has been linked to infertility and reproductive difficulties in men and women. Malnutrition, hormone abnormalities, and immune system disruptions can all have an impact on fertility, menstrual regularity, and pregnancy outcomes. Women with untreated celiac disease may have delayed menarche, irregular menstrual periods, miscarriage, and pregnancy problems.

8. Higher Risk of Specific Cancers:
Long-term untreated celiac disease increases the likelihood of developing some malignancies, including intestinal lymphoma and small intestine adenocarcinoma. Chronic inflammation and damage to the intestinal lining may contribute to the progression of malignant alterations over time, emphasizing the necessity of early detection and a gluten-free diet.

The problems of celiac disease can be severe and far-reaching if the proper diet is not followed. Individuals with celiac disease who do not strictly adhere to a gluten-free diet are more likely to experience persistent gastrointestinal symptoms, malnutrition, weight fluctuations, compromised immune function, bone disorders, neurological and psychiatric issues, infertility, and an increased risk of certain cancers. Individuals with celiac disease must work together with healthcare experts and qualified dietitians to establish and maintain a gluten-free diet that satisfies their nutritional requirements while also supporting their overall health and well-being.

Chapter 3

Meal Planning

Meal planning is an essential part of celiac disease management and a gluten-free lifestyle. Individuals with celiac disease can reduce their chance of gluten exposure by carefully arranging meals and snacks. Meal planning has various benefits for celiac disease treatment, including dietary compliance, balanced nutrition, stress and anxiety reduction, time and money savings, and promotion of general health and well-being.

The Advantages of Meal Planning for Celiac Disease Management:

1. Ensuring Dietary Compliance:

One of the key advantages of meal planning for celiac disease treatment is that it ensures nutritional compliance with a rigorous gluten-free regimen. To prevent gluten-containing foods and cross-contamination, people should plan their meals ahead of time and discover gluten-free products, recipes, and cooking techniques. This helps to avoid accidental gluten consumption while also lowering the likelihood of celiac disease symptoms and intestinal damage.

2. Maintaining Balanced Nutrition: Meal planning helps celiac patients include nutrient-rich meals to suit their nutritional demands. Individuals may ensure they acquire the vital vitamins, minerals, antioxidants, and macronutrients required for maximum health and well-being by incorporating a variety of fruits, vegetables, lean meats, gluten-free grains, and healthy fats into their meal plans.

3. Reducing Stress and Anxiety:

Following a gluten-free diet may be difficult, and uncertainty regarding food options and availability can add to stress and worry for those with celiac disease. Meal planning alleviates these worries by giving an organized approach to meal preparation while also ensuring that safe and gluten-free foods are easily available. Individuals who know what to eat and have a plan might feel more confident and empowered in managing their nutritional demands.

4. Save Time and Money:

Meal planning ahead of time may help you save time and money by eliminating the need for last-minute grocery visits, takeaway dinners, and unused items. Individuals may streamline their grocery shopping and meal preparation process by making a shopping list based on scheduled meals and storing leftovers for future meals, saving both time and money in the long term.

5. Promoting Diversity and Creativity:

Meal planning allows celiac disease patients to try new recipes, products, and cooking techniques, resulting in more diversity and creativity in their diet. By experimenting with different gluten-free grains, veggies, proteins, and spices, people may find tasty and healthy meal alternatives that keep their meals interesting and pleasurable.

6. How to Improve Portion Control and Eating Habits:

Planning meals ahead of time helps people to portion out meals and snacks based on their nutritional needs and dietary objectives. Individuals who practice portion management and mindful eating can avoid overeating, regulate their weight, and keep their blood sugar constant throughout the day.

7. Supporting Health and Wellbeing:

Overall, meal planning benefits celiac disease patients' health and well-being by encouraging adherence to a gluten-free diet, ensuring balanced nutrition, reducing stress and anxiety, saving time and money, promoting diet variety and creativity, improving portion control and eating habits, and supporting overall health and wellness.

Tips for Successful Meal Planning with Celiac Disease:

1. Begin with a Weekly Meal Plan:

Begin by planning a weekly menu that includes breakfast, lunch, supper, and snacks. When preparing meals, keep your schedule, tastes, and nutritional needs in mind, and choose a range of gluten-free dishes and ingredients to keep things exciting and balanced.

2. Check Gluten-Free Certification:

When purchasing packaged and processed goods, seek gluten-free certification marks or seals on the packaging to confirm that the items are safe for people with celiac disease. Choose certified gluten-free items wherever feasible to reduce the possibility of gluten contamination.

3. Eat entire, naturally gluten-free foods such as fruits, vegetables, lean meats, grains, legumes, nuts, and seeds. These foods are naturally gluten-free and include important nutrients for good health.

4. Batch Cooking and Preparation Ingredients:

Batch cooking and preparing items ahead of time will save you time and make meal preparation easier. Cook grains, meats, and veggies in bulk and store them in portioned containers for quick and simple meal prep throughout the week.

5. Use Leftovers Wisely: Incorporate leftovers into future dinners or repurpose them into new recipes. Leftover roasted veggies may be mixed into salads or omelets, while leftover cooked chicken can be utilized in soups or stir-fries.

6. Maintain a well-stocked pantry:

Keep a well-stocked pantry with gluten-free essentials including grains, canned beans, pasta, flour, baking ingredients, sauces, condiments, and spices. Having these ingredients on hand makes it easy to produce gluten-free meals at home.

7. Be flexible and adjust as needed.

Make your meal plan flexible and update it as required to reflect changes in your schedule, dietary choices, and item availability. If a planned dish is not practical, keep backup choices or basic meal ideas on hand to ensure that gluten-free meals are always accessible.

Meal planning is a crucial tool for controlling celiac disease and adhering to a gluten-free diet. Individuals with celiac disease who create structured meal plans can ensure dietary compliance, maintain balanced nutrition, reduce stress and anxiety, save time and money, promote variety and creativity in their diet, improve portion control and eating habits, and support overall health and well-being. Individuals with celiac disease can enjoy tasty and healthy gluten-free meals while effectively managing their illness if they prepare ahead of time.

14-day Sample Celiac Disease Meal Plan

Here's a sample 14-day meal plan for people with celiac illness that emphasizes gluten-free, nutritional, and enjoyable meals:

Day 1:

- Breakfast: Greek yogurt with fresh berries and gluten-free granola.

- Lunch: Quinoa salad with mixed veggies, chickpeas, feta cheese, and a lemon vinaigrette.

The dinner is grilled salmon with roasted sweet potatoes and steamed broccoli.

- Snack: Sliced apples and almond butter.

Day 2:

- Breakfast: Gluten-free oatmeal topped with banana slices, cinnamon, and honey.

- Lunch: Turkey and avocado lettuce wraps served with gluten-free tortilla chips and salsa.

- Dinner is gluten-free spaghetti with marinara sauce, sautéed spinach, and grilled chicken.

- Snack: Carrot sticks with hummus.

Day 3:

- Breakfast: Scrambled eggs with spinach, mushrooms, and feta cheese, served on gluten-free bread.

- Lunch: Quinoa and black bean-filled bell peppers served with mixed greens.

- Dinner: Grilled steak with roasted veggies (including bell peppers, zucchini, and onions) and quinoa.

- Snack: Greek yogurt with almond slices and honey.

Day 4:

- Breakfast: A smoothie with spinach, kale, banana, almond milk, and protein powder.

- Lunch is grilled chicken Caesar salad with gluten-free croutons and homemade Caesar dressing.

- Dinner is baked fish with quinoa pilaf and steamed asparagus.

- Snack: Rice cakes with sliced avocado and cherry tomatoes.

Day 5:

- Breakfast: Gluten-free pancakes with mixed berries and maple syrup.

- Lunch is tuna salad lettuce wraps with cucumber slices and carrot sticks.

- Dinner: Stir-fried tofu with mixed veggies and gluten-free tamari sauce on brown rice.

- Snack: Trail mix with gluten-free nuts, seeds, and dried fruit.

Day 6:

- Breakfast: Yogurt parfait layered with gluten-free granola, sliced strawberries, and honey.

- Lunch: Turkey and vegetable stir-fry with gluten-free soy sauce, served with rice noodles.

- Dinner is grilled shrimp skewers with quinoa tabbouleh and roasted cauliflower.

- Snack: Sliced pear and goat cheese on gluten-free crackers.

Day 7:

- Breakfast: A smoothie bowl topped with sliced banana, gluten-free granola, and shredded coconut.

- Lunch: Quinoa and black bean salad with avocado, cherry tomatoes, and a lime vinaigrette.

- Dinner is baked chicken breasts with mashed sweet potatoes and steamed green beans.

- Snack: Rice cakes, almond butter, and sliced strawberries.

Day 8:

- For breakfast, make gluten-free overnight oats with almond milk, chia seeds, and mixed berries.

- Lunch: Greek salad topped with grilled chicken, feta cheese, olives, cucumbers, and balsamic vinaigrette.

- Dinner is beef and veggie kebabs with quinoa pilaf and grilled corn on the cob.

- Snack: Mixture of nuts and dried fruit.

Day 9:

- Breakfast: Scrambled eggs with spinach, tomatoes, and goat cheese served on gluten-free bread.

- Lunch: Caprese salad with gluten-free croutons and a balsamic glaze.

- Dinner: Baked salmon with roasted root vegetables (carrots, parsnips, and sweet potatoes), quinoa.

- Snack: Apple slices with peanut butter.

Day 10:

- Breakfast: Gluten-free waffles topped with mixed berries and Greek yogurt.

- Lunch: turkey and avocado wraps served with gluten-free tortilla chips and salsa.

- Dinner: A vegetable stir-fry with tofu and gluten-free soy sauce served over brown rice.

- Snack: Rice cakes made with mashed avocado and cherry tomatoes.

Day 11:

- Breakfast: A smoothie with spinach, kale, pineapple, coconut milk, and protein powder.

- Lunch: A chicken Caesar salad with gluten-free croutons and homemade Caesar dressing.

The dinner is grilled steak with roasted Brussels sprouts and quinoa.

- Snack: Greek yogurt, honey, and sliced almonds.

Day 12:

- Breakfast: Gluten-free pancakes served with sliced bananas and maple syrup.

- Lunch: Tuna salad lettuce wraps with carrot and cucumber slices.

- Dinner is baked cod with quinoa pilaf and steamed broccoli.

- Snack: Trail mix with gluten-free nuts, seeds, and dried fruit.

Day 13:

- Breakfast: Yogurt parfait layered with gluten-free granola, sliced strawberries, and honey.

- Lunch: Quinoa and black bean salad with avocado, cherry tomatoes, and a lime vinaigrette.

The dinner is grilled shrimp skewers with roasted sweet potatoes and green beans.

- Snack: Sliced pear and goat cheese on gluten-free crackers.

Day 14:

- Breakfast: A smoothie bowl topped with mixed berries, gluten-free granola, and shredded coconut.
- Lunch: Greek salad topped with grilled chicken, feta cheese, olives, cucumbers, and balsamic vinaigrette.
- Dinner: Beef and vegetable stir-fry with gluten-free soy sauce served with rice noodles.
- Snack: Mixture of nuts and dried fruit.

This 14-day meal plan includes a range of gluten-free breakfast, lunch, supper, and snack options to assist celiac disease patients eat tasty and healthy meals while efficiently managing their illness. It focuses on entire, naturally gluten-free foods and contains a mix of proteins, carbs, healthy fats, fruits, and vegetables to support general health.

Instructions

Here are the steps for following the 14-day food plan:

1. Review the food Plan: Spend some time reviewing the 14-day food plan given. Familiarize yourself with the daily breakfast, lunch, dinner, and snack offerings.

2. Check the Ingredients: Go over each day of the meal plan and look for any ingredients you might need to buy. Make a note of anything you don't already have in your cupboard or refrigerator.

3. Go grocery shopping. Go to the grocery shop with your list of ingredients. If you're on a celiac disease diet, look for gluten-free alternatives to staples like bread, pasta, and flour.

4. Meal Prep: Before beginning the meal plan, consider completing some meal prep to save time over the week. This may entail washing and cutting vegetables, cooking grains such as rice or quinoa, and preparing sauces or dressings.

5. Follow the Plan: Each day, adhere to the eating plan as specified. Start your day with a nutritious breakfast, eat filling lunches and dinners, and add healthy snacks as required to stay energized throughout the day.

6. Stay Hydrated: Drink lots of water throughout the day to keep yourself hydrated. For a little more taste, try herbal teas or infused water.

7. Listen to Your Body: Pay attention to how your body feels when following the dietary plan. If you find yourself hungry in between meals, you may need to alter your portion sizes or include an extra snack.

8. Modify as needed:. Feel free to change the meal plan to accommodate your tastes, dietary constraints, or food allergies. You may change the components, tweak the portion proportions, or substitute different meals entirely.

9. Be Consistent: Consistency is essential while following a food plan. Stick to the plan as strictly as possible to get the full advantages of healthy eating and maintain a balanced diet.

10. Enjoy the Process: Throughout the 14-day meal plan, take advantage of the chance to experiment with new dishes and flavors. Cooking and eating healthful meals may be an enjoyable and rewarding experience!

Following these guidelines will allow you to effectively apply the 14-day meal plan and enjoy a range of tasty and healthy gluten-free meals. Remember to listen to your body, remain hydrated, and modify the diet as necessary to meet your requirements and preferences.

Chapter 4

Essential Equipment and Items

Creating a celiac disease cookbook necessitates several tools and supplies to guarantee that the recipes are properly prepared and presented. Here's a checklist of essentials:

1. Cookware: - Nonstick frying pan

- Saucepans in various sizes.

- Baking sheet and pan

- Casserole dishes.

- Stockpot for soups and stews.

2. kitchen utensils:

- Chef's and paring knives.

- Cutting Board

- Mixing Bowls

- A whisk

- wooden spoons and spatulas.

- Measuring cup and spoon

- Rolling pin for gluten-free baking.

- Pastry Brush

- Grater - Kitchen scale.

3. Appliances:

- Oven - Stovetop - Blender/food processor - Stand mixer or hand mixer (for baking)

- Toaster for gluten-free bread.

4. Specialized Equipment: - Bread machine (for gluten-free bread)

- Pasta maker (gluten-free pasta).

- Rice Cooker

- Slow cooker or Instant Pot (for easy cooking).

5. Food Storage: - Use airtight containers for ingredients and freezer-safe containers for leftovers for batch cooking.

6. Other Item:

- Recipe notebook or computer for recipe creation and organization.

- Use a camera or smartphone to photograph recipes.

- Food styling props, such as plates, utensils, and napkins.

- Kitchen towels, oven mitts.

- Apron to protect garments while cooking.

7. ingredients:

- Gluten-free flour (such as almond flour, coconut flour, and rice flour).

- Gluten-free grains (such as quinoa, millet, and buckwheat).

- Gluten-free carbohydrates (such as potato starch, tapioca starch, and cornstarch).

- Gluten-free baking ingredients (xanthan gum, baking powder, baking soda, etc.)

- Fresh fruit and veggies.

- Lean proteins, such as chicken, turkey, fish, and tofu.

- Dairy-free options (such as almond milk, coconut milk, and dairy-free cheese).

- Herbs, spices, and seasoning

With this equipment and ingredients, you will be able to make tasty and safe dishes for people with celiac disease, allowing them to enjoy a diverse range of flavorful and gratifying meals.

Day 1:

Breakfast: Greek Yogurt Parfait.

Ingredients: -1 cup Greek yogurt

- 1/2 cup gluten-free granola.

Add 1/2 cup mixed berries (strawberries, blueberries, raspberries) and 1 tablespoon honey (optional).

- Instructions:

1. In a glass or dish, combine the Greek yogurt, gluten-free granola, and mixed berries.

2. Repeat the layers until all of the ingredients have been used up.

3. Drizzle with honey if desired.

4. Serve immediately and enjoy!

Lunch: Quinoa Salad.

Ingredients: 1 cup cooked quinoa, 1/2 cup diced cucumber, 1/2 cup split cherry tomatoes, 1/4 cup diced red onion, 1/4 cup crumbled feta cheese, 2 teaspoons minced fresh parsley, and 2 tablespoons lemon juice.

- One tablespoon of olive oil.

- Add salt and pepper to taste.

- Instructions:

1. In a large mixing bowl, add cooked quinoa, cucumber, cherry tomatoes, red onion, feta cheese, and parsley.

2. In a small bowl, combine the lemon juice, olive oil, salt, and pepper.

3. Pour the dressing over the quinoa and toss to incorporate.

4. Serve chilled or at room temperature.

Dinner: Grilled salmon

Ingredients: 4 salmon fillets, 2 tablespoons olive oil, and 2 chopped garlic cloves.

Ingredients: 1 teaspoon lemon zest, 1 tablespoon lemon juice.

- Season to taste with salt and pepper. - Instructions:

1. Preheat the grill to medium-high heat.

2. In a small bowl, combine the olive oil, garlic, lemon zest, lemon juice, salt, and pepper.

3. Brush the marinade over the salmon fillets on both sides.

4. Grill the salmon for 4-5 minutes per side, or until it flakes easily with a fork.

5. Serve hot, with your choice of sides.

snack: sliced apples with almond butter

Ingredients: - One sliced apple.

- Two tablespoons of almond butter.

- Instructions:

1. Spread almond butter onto apple slices.

2. Enjoy a tasty and healthy snack!

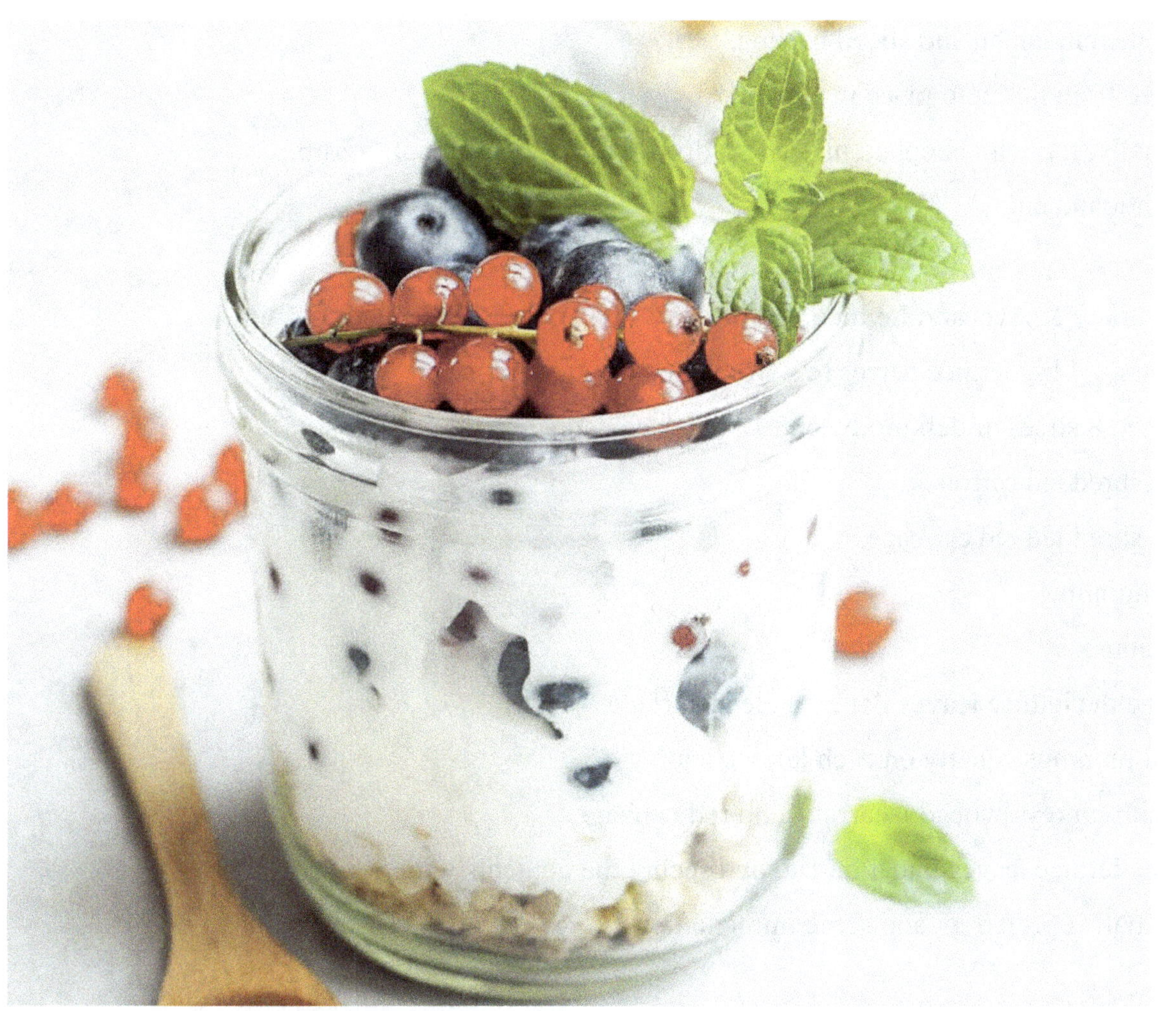

Day 2:

Breakfast: Gluten-free oatmeal

Ingredients: - 1/2 cup gluten-free oatmeal

- One cup of almond milk.

-1/2 teaspoon cinnamon

- 1/2 banana, cut

- 1 tablespoon of chopped nuts (optional).

- One teaspoon of honey or maple syrup (optional)

- Instructions:

1. In a small saucepan, mix gluten-free oats and almond milk.

2. Bring to a simmer over medium heat, stirring regularly.

3. Cook for 5-7 minutes, or until oats are cooked and the mixture thickens.

4. Stir in the cinnamon and sliced banana.

5. Remove from heat and place in a dish.

6. Optionally, top with chopped nuts and a drizzle of honey or maple syrup.

7. Serve hot and enjoy!

Lunch: Turkey & Avocado Lettuce Wraps

Ingredients: - 4 big lettuce leaves (e.g. romaine or butter lettuce).

Ingredients: 8 slices of deli turkey and 1 sliced avocado.

- 1/2 cup shredded carrots.

- 1/2 cup shredded red cabbage.

-1/4 cup hummus

- Instructions:

1. Arrange the lettuce leaves flat on a clean surface.

2. Spread hummus equally on each lettuce leaf.

3. Top with turkey, avocado, carrots, and red cabbage.

4. Roll the lettuce leaves into a burrito and secure the contents within.

5. Cut in half if preferred, and serve immediately.

Dinner: gluten-free pasta with marinara sauce

Ingredients: - 8 oz gluten-free pasta - 2 cups marinara sauce (either store-bought or homemade)

- Fresh basil leaves as garnish

- Grated Parmesan cheese is optional.

- Instructions:

1. Cook the gluten-free pasta according to the package directions.

2. Drain the pasta and return it to the saucepan.

3. In a separate pot, heat the marinara sauce until it is warmed through.

4. Pour marinara sauce over cooked spaghetti and toss to coat.

5. Arrange the spaghetti on serving dishes and decorate them with fresh basil leaves.

6. If preferred, garnish with grated Parmesan cheese and serve hot.

Snack: Carrot sticks and hummus

Ingredients: - 2 big peeled carrots sliced into sticks.

-1/4 cup hummus

Instructions: 1. Pair carrot sticks with hummus for a crisp and delicious snack.

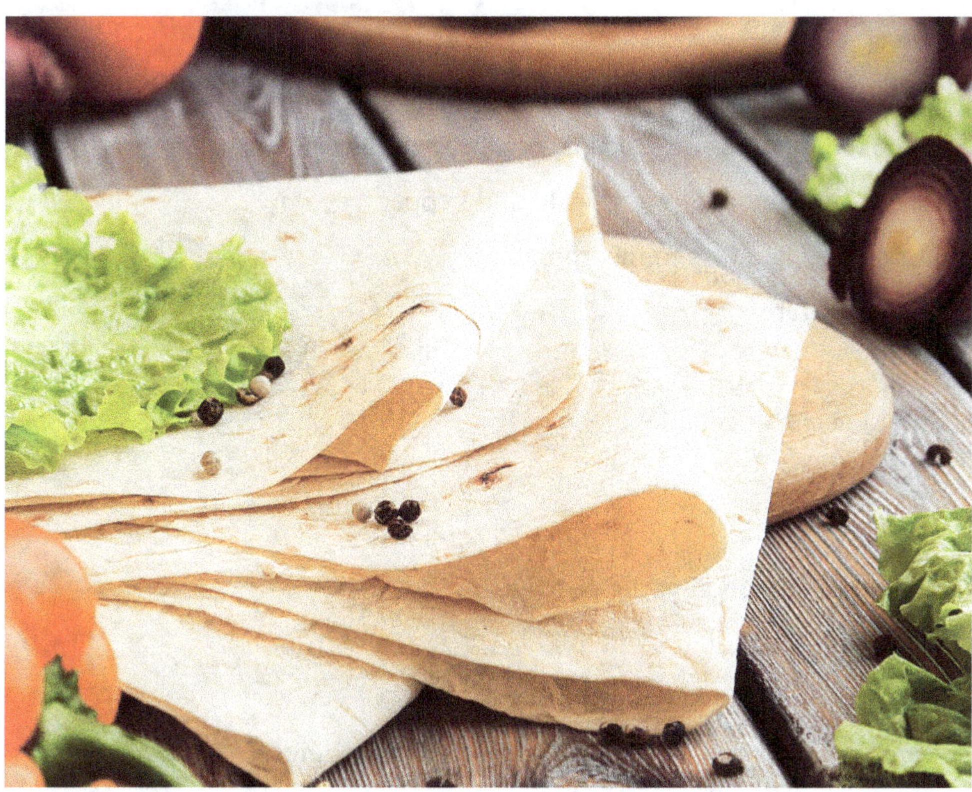

Day 3:

Breakfast: Scrambled Eggs with Spinach and Feta.

Ingredients: - Four eggs.

Ingredients: 1/4 cup milk, 1 cup fresh spinach leaves, and 1/4 cup crumbled feta cheese.

- Season to taste with salt and pepper. - Instructions:

1. Whisk the eggs and milk together in a mixing basin until thoroughly blended.

2. Heat a nonstick skillet over medium heat, then add the egg mixture.

3. Cook, stirring periodically, until the eggs are nearly set.

4. Add the spinach leaves and simmer until they wilt and the eggs are thoroughly cooked.

5. Remove from heat and sprinkle with crumbled feta cheese.

6. Serve hot and enjoy!

Lunch: Quinoa & Black Bean Salad

Ingredients: 1 cup cooked quinoa and 1 cup rinsed and drained black beans.

- Add 1/2 cup sliced bell pepper and 1/4 cup minced cilantro.

- 2 teaspoons of lime juice.

- One tablespoon of olive oil.

- Season to taste with salt and pepper. - Instructions:

1. In a large bowl, mix the cooked quinoa, black beans, bell pepper, and cilantro.

2. In a small bowl, combine the lime juice, olive oil, salt, and pepper.

3. Pour the dressing over the quinoa and toss to incorporate.

4. Serve chilled or at room temperature.

Dinner: Grilled Chicken and Roasted Vegetables

Ingredients:

- Four chicken breasts.

- Add 2 tablespoons olive oil and 1 teaspoon garlic powder.

- One teaspoon of paprika.

- 1/2 teaspoon dried thyme.

- Season with salt and pepper to taste. - Add 2 cups of mixed veggies (e.g., bell peppers, zucchini, onions).

- Instructions:

1. Preheat the grill to medium-high heat.

2. In a small bowl, mix olive oil, garlic powder, paprika, dried thyme, salt, and pepper.

3. Rub the spice mixture onto the chicken breasts.

4. Grill the chicken for 6-8 minutes per side, or until well done and no longer pink in the center.

5. Meanwhile, stir the veggies with olive oil, salt, and pepper.

6. Grill the veggies for 8-10 minutes, or until they are soft and gently browned.

7. Serve grilled chicken alongside roasted veggies.

Snack: Rice Cakes With Almond Butter And Banana

Ingredients: - Two rice cakes.

Ingredients: 2 tablespoons almond butter and 1 sliced banana.

- Instructions:

1. Spread almond butter evenly on rice cakes.

2. Top with sliced bananas.

3. Eat as a satisfying snack!

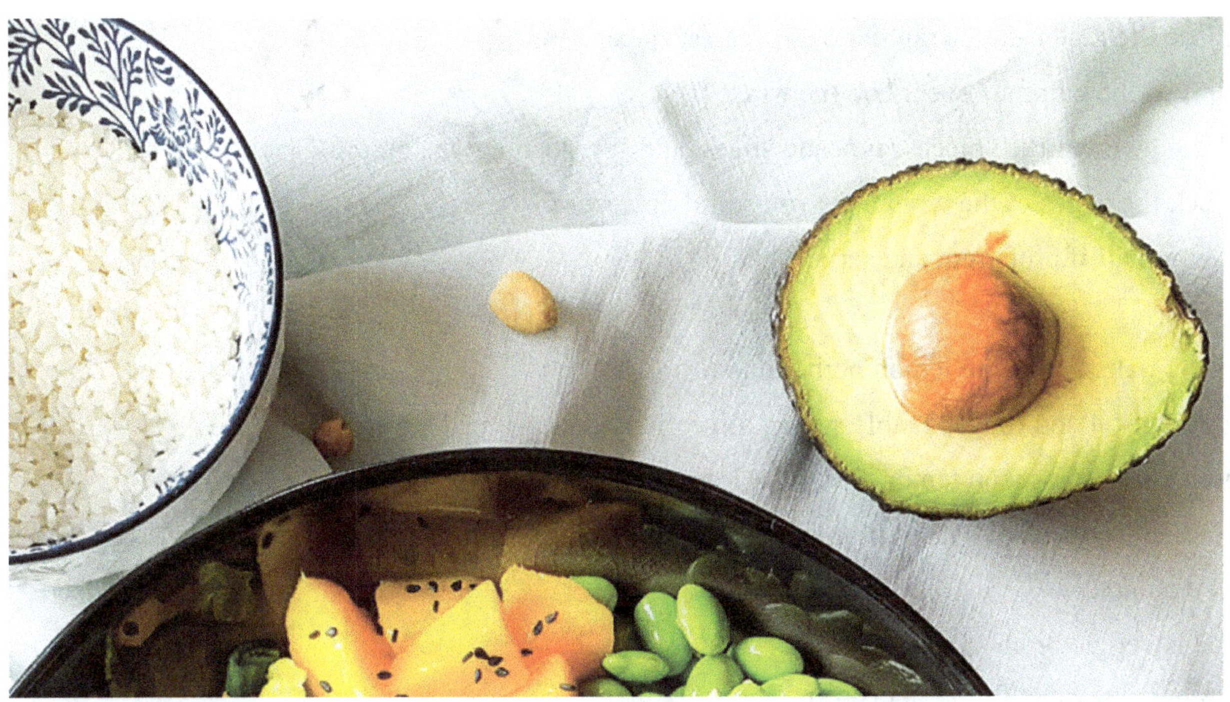

Day 4:

Breakfast: Smoothie bowl

Ingredients: - One frozen banana.

- 1/2 cup frozen mixed berries.

-1/2 cup spinach leaves

- One-half cup almond milk

Toppings include sliced banana, granola, chia seeds, and shredded coconut.

- Instructions:

1. In a blender, combine the frozen banana, mixed berries, spinach, and almond milk.

2. Blend until smooth and creamy.

3. Transfer to a bowl and top with sliced bananas, granola, chia seeds, and shredded coconut.

4. Enjoy with a spoon!

Lunch: Turkey & Avocado Wrap

Ingredients: - One gluten-free wrap - Three slices of deli turkey - 1/4 sliced avocado

- 1/4 cup shredded lettuce.

- 1 tbsp hummus - Directions:

1. Place the gluten-free wrap flat on a clean surface.

2. Spread the hummus evenly on the wrap.

3. Arrange the turkey pieces, avocado slices, and shredded lettuce on top.

4. Tuck the edges of the wrap in as you roll it up securely.

5. Cut in half if preferred, and serve.

Dinner: Baked cod with lemon herb quinoa

Ingredients: 4 cod fillets, 2 tablespoons olive oil, and 2 chopped garlic cloves.

Ingredients: 1 teaspoon lemon zest, 1 tablespoon lemon juice.

Ingredients: 1 teaspoon dried thyme, 1 teaspoon dried parsley, salt and pepper to taste, and 1 cup rinsed quinoa.

- 2 cups veggie broth - Directions:

1. Preheat the oven to 375°F (190° C).

2. In a small mixing bowl, combine olive oil, garlic, lemon zest, lemon juice, dried thyme, dried parsley, salt, and pepper.

3. Put the cod fillets on a baking tray and brush with the olive oil mixture.

4. Bake cod in a preheated oven for 15-20 minutes, or until it is opaque and readily flaked with a fork.

5. Meanwhile, bring vegetable broth to a boil in a saucepan.

6. Stir in the quinoa, then decrease the heat to low, cover, and simmer for 15-20 minutes, or until the quinoa is cooked and the liquid has been absorbed.

7. Fluff quinoa with a fork before serving with baked cod.

Snack: Greek Yogurt and Berries

Ingredients: - 1/2 cup Greek yogurt.

- 1/4 cup mixed berries (strawberries, raspberries, blueberries)

- One spoonful of honey (optional).

- Instructions:

1. In a dish, combine the Greek yogurt and mixed berries.

2. Drizzle with honey if desired.

3. Eat as a refreshing snack!

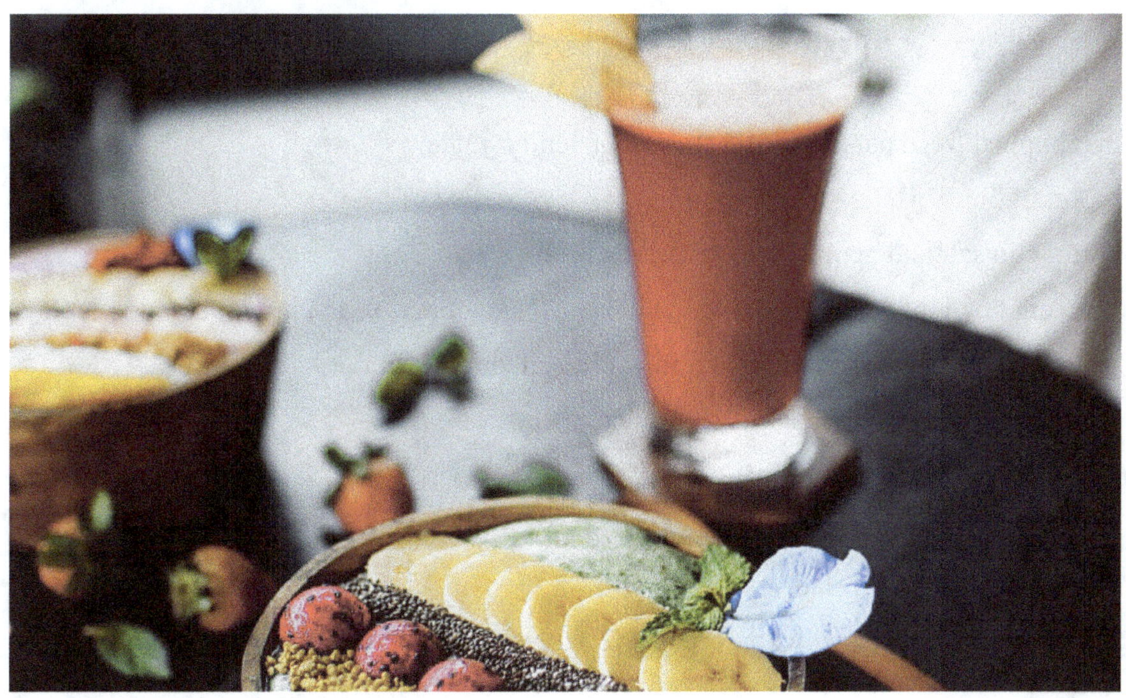

Day 5:

Breakfast: Gluten-free pancakes

Ingredients include 1 cup gluten-free flour, 1 tablespoon sugar, and 1 teaspoon baking powder.

- One-half teaspoon baking soda

- 1/4 tsp salt - 1 cup almond milk.

Ingredients: 2 tablespoons melted coconut oil, 1 teaspoon vanilla essence.

- Instructions:

1. In a large basin, combine gluten-free flour, sugar, baking powder, baking soda, and salt.

2. In a separate dish, combine the almond milk, melted coconut oil, and vanilla essence.

3. Pour the wet ingredients into the dry ingredients and whisk just until incorporated.

4. Heat a nonstick pan over medium heat and gently coat it with coconut oil.

5. Pour batter into the skillet to make pancakes.

6. Cook until bubbles appear on the top, then turn and cook until golden brown on the opposite side.

7. Serve hot with your preferred toppings.

Lunch: Quinoa and Chickpea Salad.

Ingredients:

- 1 cup cooked quinoa, 1 cup cooked chickpeas, 1/2 diced cucumber, and 1/2 diced red bell pepper.

- Add 1/4 cup chopped fresh parsley and 2 teaspoons lemon juice.

- One tablespoon of olive oil.

- Season to taste with salt and pepper. - Instructions:

1. In a large mixing bowl, add cooked quinoa, chickpeas, cucumber, red bell pepper, and parsley.

2. In a small bowl, combine the lemon juice, olive oil, salt, and pepper.

3. Pour the dressing over the quinoa and toss to incorporate.

4. Serve chilled or at room temperature.

Dinner: Grilled chicken Caesar salad

Ingredients: 2 boneless, skinless chicken breasts, 2 tablespoons olive oil, and 1 teaspoon garlic powder.

- one teaspoon dried oregano.

- Add salt and pepper to taste. - Chop 6 cups of romaine lettuce.

- Use 1/4 cup grated Parmesan cheese and 1/2 cup gluten-free croutons.

- Caesar dressing, store-bought or homemade.

- Instructions:

1. Preheat the grill to medium-high heat.

2. In a small bowl, combine olive oil, garlic powder, dried oregano, salt, and pepper.

3. Coat the chicken breasts with the olive oil mixture.

4. Grill the chicken for 6-8 minutes on each side, or until well done.

5. Let the chicken rest for a few minutes before slicing thinly.

6. In a large mixing bowl, add chopped romaine lettuce, sliced grilled chicken, Parmesan cheese, and gluten-free croutons.

7. Toss in Caesar dressing until evenly covered.

8. Serve immediately and enjoy!

Snack: Rice Cake with Peanut Butter

Ingredients: - One rice cake - Two teaspoons of peanut butter

- Instructions:

1. Spread peanut butter over the rice cake.

2. Enjoy a fast and filling snack.

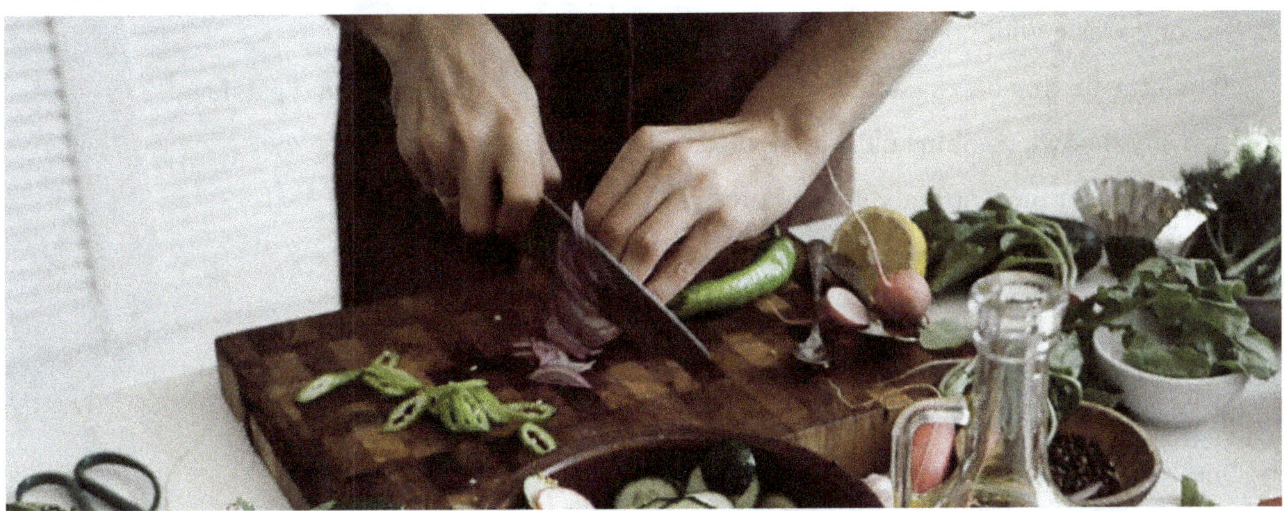

Day 6:

Breakfast: Chia Seed Pudding.

Ingredients: -1/4 cup chia seeds

- One cup of almond milk.

- One tablespoon of honey or maple syrup (optional)

Toppings include sliced strawberries, almonds, and shredded coconut. Add 1/2 teaspoon vanilla extract.

- Instructions:

1. In a dish, combine the chia seeds, almond milk, honey or maple syrup (if using), and vanilla essence.

2. Cover and refrigerate for at least 2 hours, preferably overnight, to thicken.

3. Before serving, stir thoroughly and garnish with sliced strawberries, almonds, and shredded coconut.

4. Serve cold for a tasty and nutritious breakfast!

Lunch: Lentil salad

Ingredients: 1 cup cooked lentils and 1/2 chopped cucumber.

- 1/2 red onion, diced.

- Add 1/4 cup chopped fresh parsley and 2 teaspoons lemon juice.

- One tablespoon of olive oil.

- Season to taste with salt and pepper. - Instructions:

1. In a large mixing bowl, add the cooked lentils, cucumber, red onion, and parsley.

2. In a small bowl, combine the lemon juice, olive oil, salt, and pepper.

3. Toss together the lentil mixture and dressing.

4. Serve chilled or at room temperature.

Dinner: Gluten-free Pizza

Ingredients: - One gluten-free pizza dough (store-bought or handmade).

- One-half cup pizza sauce

- One cup of shredded mozzarella cheese

- Add your favorite toppings, such as sliced bell peppers, mushrooms, olives, tomatoes, cooked chicken, and so on.

- Instructions:

1. Preheat the oven to 425°F (220°C).

2. Transfer the gluten-free pizza dough to a baking sheet lined with parchment paper.

3. Spread the pizza sauce evenly on the crust, leaving a little border around the borders.

4. Sprinkle the sauce with shredded mozzarella cheese.

5. Spread your preferred toppings over the cheese.

6. Cook the pizza in the preheated oven for 12-15 minutes, or until the cheese is melted and bubbling.

7. Slice and serve hot.

Snack: Trail Mix.

Ingredients: - 1/2 cup gluten-free nuts (such as almonds, cashews, or walnuts).

- 1/4 cup gluten-free seeds (pumpkin or sunflower seeds)

- 1/4 cup dried fruit (such as raisins, cranberries, or apricots)

- Instructions:

1. Combine gluten-free nuts, seeds, and dried fruit in a dish.

2. Separate into separate servings for an easy on-the-go snack.

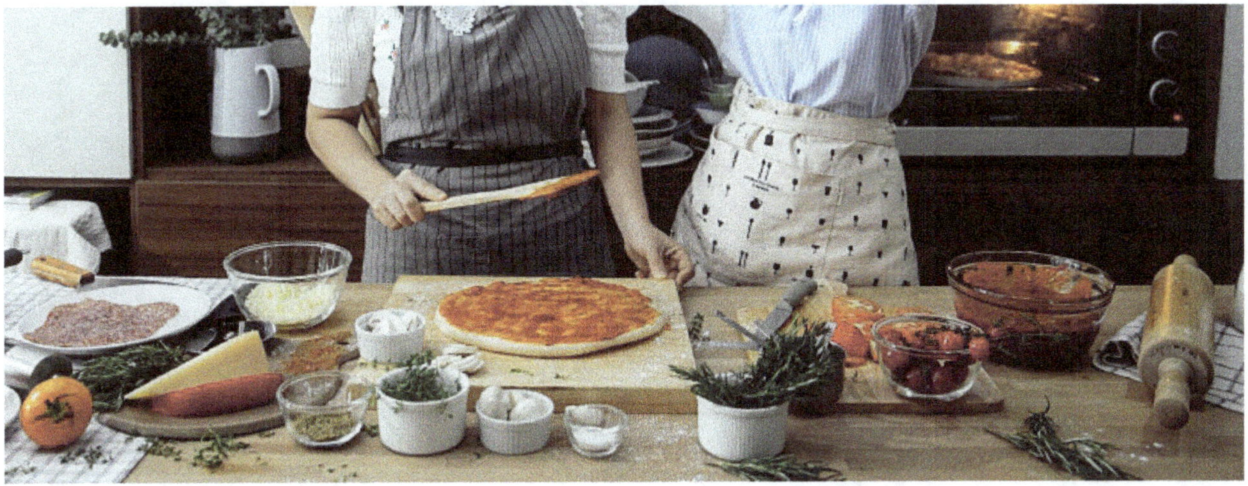

Day 7:

Breakfast: Banana Almond Butter Toast.

Ingredients: 2 slices gluten-free bread, 2 tablespoons almond butter, and 1 sliced banana.

- One spoonful of honey (optional).

- Instructions:

1. Toast the gluten-free bread until golden brown.

2. Spread almond butter equally on each slice of bread.

3. Top with sliced bananas.

4. Add honey if desired.

5. Enjoy a simple and filling breakfast!

Lunch: Caprese salad

Ingredients: - 2 big, sliced tomatoes.

- 1 ball fresh mozzarella cheese, sliced

- Fresh basil leaves - Balsamic glaze.

- Season to taste with salt and pepper. - Instructions:

1. Arrange tomato and mozzarella slices on a serving dish in alternate order.

2. Tuck fresh basil leaves between the tomato and mozzarella pieces.

3. Drizzle with balsamic glaze.

4. Season with salt and pepper, to taste.

5. Serve immediately for a refreshing lunch choice.

Dinner: beef stir-fry with rice

Ingredients: - 1 lb thinly sliced beef sirloin - 2 teaspoons gluten-free soy sauce.

- One tablespoon of sesame oil.

- 2 garlic cloves, minced

- 1 tablespoon of minced ginger

- 1 onion, sliced

- 1 bell pepper, cut

- One cup of broccoli florets.

- Cooked rice to serve

- Instructions:

1. In a bowl, combine the sliced beef, gluten-free soy sauce, and sesame oil. Set aside for 15-20 minutes.

2. Preheat a wok or big pan to high heat.

3. Stir in the minced garlic and ginger, cooking for 30 seconds.

4. Stir-fry the marinated beef slices until browned and well done.

5. Add the chopped onion, bell pepper, and broccoli florets to the wok and stir-fry until the veggies are soft and crisp.

6. Serve the beef stir-fry hot with prepared rice.

Snack: Rice Crackers and Guacamole

Ingredients: 6 rice crackers and 1 ripe avocado.

- One tablespoon of lime juice.

- Season to taste with salt and pepper. - Instructions:

1. In a bowl, mash the ripe avocado with the lime juice until smooth.

2. Add salt and pepper to taste.

3. Serve rice crackers with guacamole for a tasty and filling snack.

You can change the recipes to suit your taste preferences and dietary requirements. Enjoy your meals!

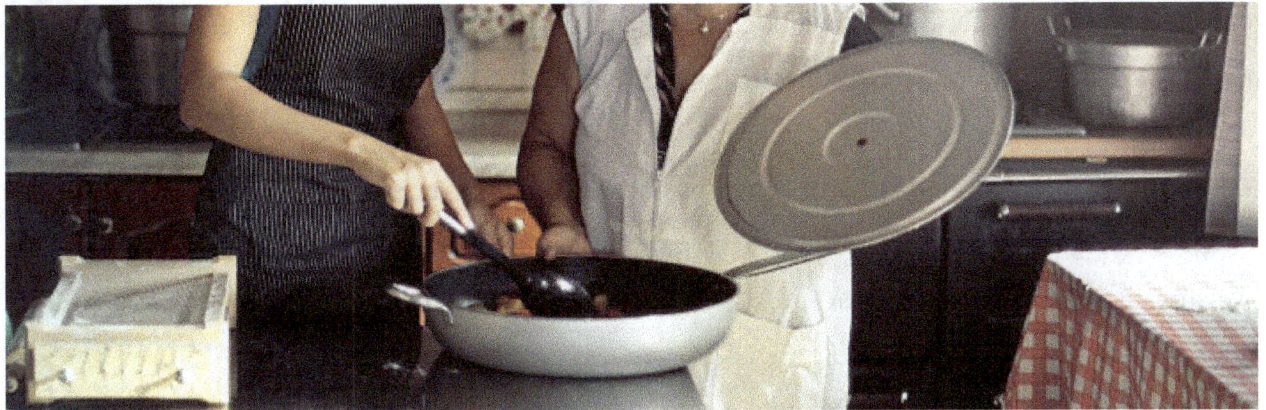

Timing Your Meal

Individuals with celiac disease must adhere to eating schedules and meal planning to manage symptoms and preserve general health. Here are some meal timings for celiac disease patients:

1. Consistency: Eating meals and snacks at regular intervals throughout the day can help control blood sugar levels and reduce hunger-induced food choices that include gluten. Aim for three balanced meals and one to two snacks each day.

2. Timing for Gluten-Free Meals: Gluten-containing foods can cause symptoms in people with celiac disease, so it's vital to prepare gluten-free meals and snacks. Make sure you thoroughly check all components and food products for gluten.

3. Prep Time: Allow yourself extra time to make gluten-free meals and snacks, especially if you're cooking from scratch or experimenting with new recipes. This can assist to minimize stress and ensure that you always have healthful alternatives accessible.

4. Post-meal activities: Some people with celiac disease may feel fatigued or uncomfortable after eating, especially if they accidentally absorbed gluten. Consider arranging less taxing activities or setting aside time for rest after meals.

5. Hydration: Remember to remain hydrated during the day by drinking lots of water. Adequate hydration is essential for digestion and general health, particularly for celiac disease patients who may have diarrhea or other gastrointestinal symptoms.

6. Mindful Eating: Practice mindful eating by focusing on hunger and fullness indicators, as well as the sensory experience of eating. This can assist to reduce overeating and increase meal pleasure.

7. Meal Time and Medication: If you take medicine for celiac disease or similar illnesses, such as vitamin supplements or digestive enzymes, make sure to time your meals and medications correctly to promote maximum absorption and efficacy.

8. Plad: Plan your meals and snacks ahead of time to ensure that gluten-free choices are accessible, especially if you're eating out or traveling. Bring gluten-free snacks or dinners if necessary to prevent being left without safe food alternatives.

Individuals with celiac disease can effectively control their symptoms, improve their general health, and enjoy a gratifying and pleasant dining experience by adhering to a gluten-free diet and paying attention to meal times.

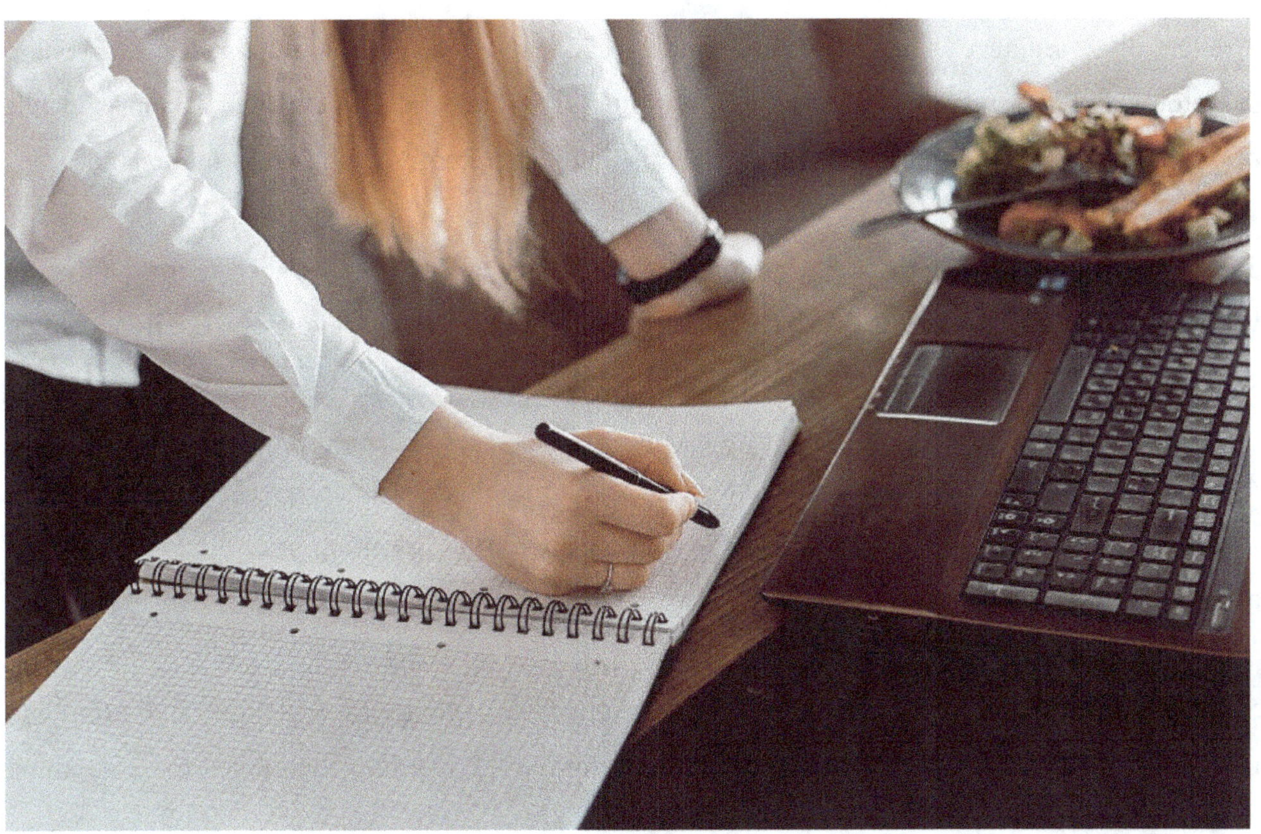

Hydration

Hydration is crucial for everyone, including celiac patients. Proper hydration improves digestion, nutrition absorption, and general health. Here are several hydration considerations for people with celiac disease:

1. Water intake: Adequate water consumption is critical for celiac disease patients, especially if they have gastrointestinal symptoms like diarrhea or vomiting. Drinking enough water helps to avoid dehydration and maintain optimum hydration levels.

2. Electrolyte Balance: Diarrhea and vomiting can cause electrolyte imbalances, worsening symptoms and affecting general health. Consuming electrolyte-rich fluids, such as sports drinks or oral rehydration treatments, can aid in replenishing lost electrolytes and restoring balance.

3. Gluten-free Drinks: Be aware of gluten-containing substances in beverages such as flavored waters, sodas, and sports drinks. Choose gluten-free choices to avoid inadvertent gluten exposure.

4. Limit Caffeine and Alcohol: Caffeinated and alcoholic beverages can have a diuretic impact, leading to increased fluid loss and perhaps greater dehydration. Limiting your intake of caffeine and alcohol might help you stay hydrated.

5. Herbal Teas: Celiac disease patients might benefit from herbal teas, which are hydrating and relaxing. Choose gluten-free herbal teas like chamomile, peppermint, or ginger for a soothing and hydrating beverage.

6. Fruits and vegetables: Add hydrating fruits and vegetables to your diet, such as watermelon, cucumber, oranges, and strawberries. These meals contain a lot of water and help keep you hydrated.

7. Monitor the symptoms: Pay attention to symptoms of dehydration, such as dark urine, dry mouth, weariness, and dizziness. If you have these symptoms, drink more fluids and try electrolyte-rich drinks to help you rehydrate.

8. Hydration During Exercise: Drink plenty of water before, during, and after your workout. Consider replacing electrolytes lost via perspiration with sports drinks or electrolyte pills.

9. Travel Considerations: When traveling, especially in locations where clean drinking water may be scarce, bring a reusable water container and replenish it with bottled or treated water from reliable sources.

Individuals suffering from celiac disease can improve their overall health, control symptoms, and maintain optimal well-being by emphasizing hydration and selecting hydrating beverages and foods. Remember to drink water throughout the day and vary fluid intake to meet individual needs and activity levels.

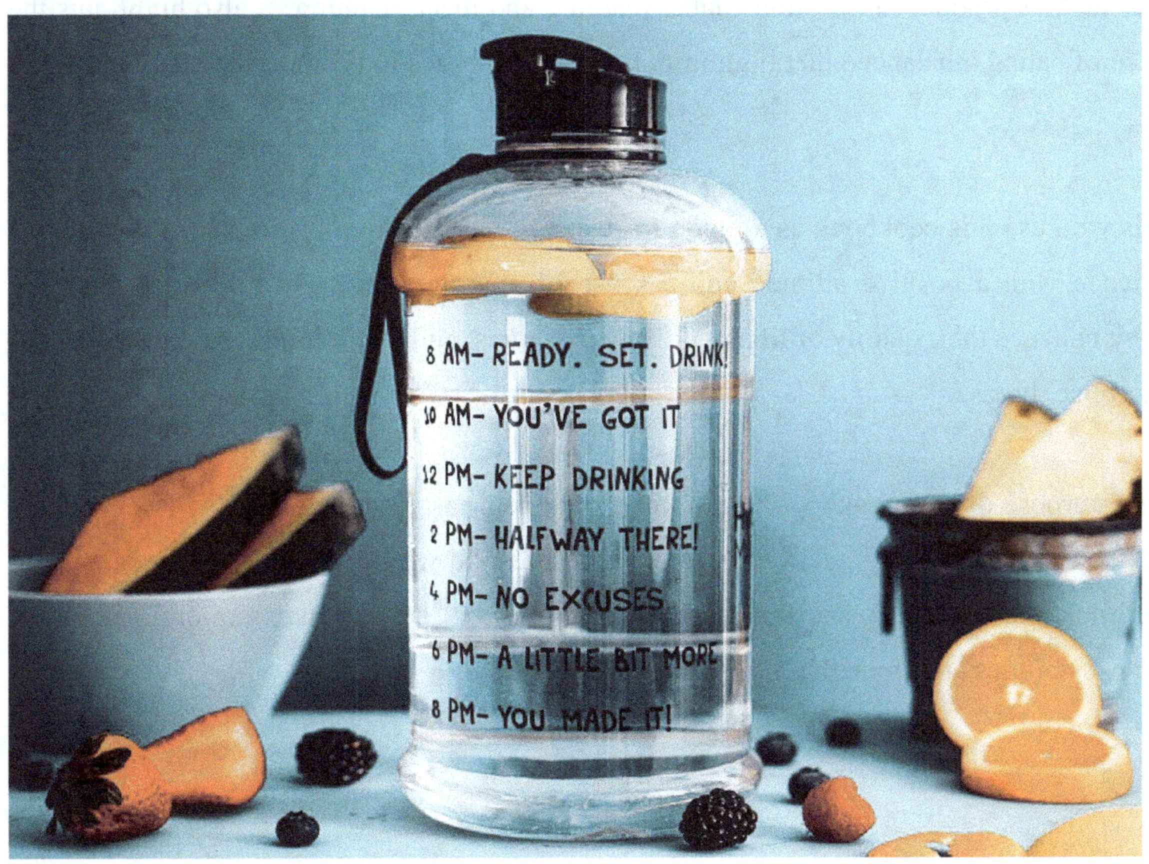

Conclusion

Finally, this celiac illness cookbook provides a thorough guide to living well with gluten sensitivity and celiac disease. This cookbook encourages people to take charge of their health and adopt a gluten-free lifestyle by giving a variety of tasty and nutritious recipes, as well as essential information on celiac disease, its causes, symptoms, and management techniques.

This cookbook contains unique and fulfilling recipes that cater to a wide range of tastes and dietary needs, from robust breakfast alternatives to tasty main courses and luscious desserts. Each dish is meticulously designed to be gluten-free, guaranteeing that people with celiac disease may eat meals that are not only safe but also pleasurable and satisfying.

Beyond the recipes, this cookbook provides practical advice for handling the problems of gluten-free living, such as product substitutions, label reading, and meal planning. It also highlights the significance of eating a balanced diet high in nutrient-dense foods to promote general health and well-being.

Individuals who use this cookbook as a guide for their gluten-free journey are urged to embrace the experience with a positive attitude and a sense of empowerment. By following this diet, readers may enhance their quality of life, decrease symptoms, and avoid long-term consequences caused by celiac disease.

Finally, the purpose of this cookbook is not only to present tasty recipes but also to encourage and push people to accept and adapt to a gluten-free lifestyle with confidence and excitement. With determination, ingenuity, and the help of this cookbook, readers may explore a world of delectable possibilities and flourish on their gluten-free journey.

Weekly Meal PLANNER

DATE ___ / ___ / ___

MONDAY

Breakfast

Lunch

Dinner

Snack

TUESDAY

Breakfast

Lunch

Dinner

Snack

WEDNESDAY

Breakfast

Lunch

Dinner

Snack

THURSDAY

Breakfast

Lunch

Dinner

Snack

FRIDAY

Breakfast

Lunch

Dinner

Snack

SATURDAY

Breakfast

Lunch

Dinner

Snack

SUNDAY

Breakfast

Lunch

Dinner

Snack

WATER INTAKE

MONDAY							
TUESDAY							
WEDNESDAY							
THURSDAY							
FRIDAY							
SATURDAY							
SUNDAY							

CELIAC DISEASE COOKBOOK

Weekly Meal PLANNER

DATE ___ / ___ / ___

MONDAY

Breakfast |

Lunch |

Dinner |

Snack |

TUESDAY

Breakfast |

Lunch |

Dinner |

Snack |

WEDNESDAY

Breakfast |

Lunch |

Dinner |

Snack |

THURSDAY

Breakfast |

Lunch |

Dinner |

Snack |

FRIDAY

Breakfast |

Lunch |

Dinner |

Snack |

SATURDAY

Breakfast |

Lunch |

Dinner |

Snack |

SUNDAY

Breakfast |

Lunch |

Dinner |

Snack |

WATER INTAKE

MONDAY	
TUESDAY	
WEDNESDAY	
THURSDAY	
FRIDAY	
SATURDAY	
SUNDAY	

CELIAC DISEASE COOKBOOK

Weekly Meal PLANNER

DATE ___/___/___

MONDAY

Breakfast |

Lunch |

Dinner |

Snack |

TUESDAY

Breakfast |

Lunch |

Dinner |

Snack |

WEDNESDAY

Breakfast |

Lunch |

Dinner |

Snack |

THURSDAY

Breakfast |

Lunch |

Dinner |

Snack |

FRIDAY

Breakfast |

Lunch |

Dinner |

Snack |

SATURDAY

Breakfast |

Lunch |

Dinner |

Snack |

SUNDAY

Breakfast |

Lunch |

Dinner |

Snack |

WATER INTAKE

MONDAY									
TUESDAY									
WEDNESDAY									
THURSDAY									
FRIDAY									
SATURDAY									
SUNDAY									

CELIAC DISEASE COOKBOOK

Weekly Meal PLANNER

DATE ___/___/___

MONDAY

Breakfast |
Lunch |
Dinner |
Snack |

TUESDAY

Breakfast |
Lunch |
Dinner |
Snack |

WEDNESDAY

Breakfast |
Lunch |
Dinner |
Snack |

THURSDAY

Breakfast |
Lunch |
Dinner |
Snack |

FRIDAY

Breakfast |
Lunch |
Dinner |
Snack |

SATURDAY

Breakfast |
Lunch |
Dinner |
Snack |

SUNDAY

Breakfast |
Lunch |
Dinner |
Snack |

WATER INTAKE

| MONDAY |
| TUESDAY |
| WEDNESDAY |
| THURSDAY |
| FRIDAY |
| SATURDAY |
| SUNDAY |

CELIAC DISEASE COOKBOOK

Weekly Meal PLANNER

DATE ___ / ___ / ___

MONDAY

Breakfast |

Lunch |

Dinner |

Snack |

TUESDAY

Breakfast |

Lunch |

Dinner |

Snack |

WEDNESDAY

Breakfast |

Lunch |

Dinner |

Snack |

THURSDAY

Breakfast |

Lunch |

Dinner |

Snack |

FRIDAY

Breakfast |

Lunch |

Dinner |

Snack |

SATURDAY

Breakfast |

Lunch |

Dinner |

Snack |

SUNDAY

Breakfast |

Lunch |

Dinner |

Snack |

WATER INTAKE									
MONDAY									
TUESDAY									
WEDNESDAY									
THURSDAY									
FRIDAY									
SATURDAY									
SUNDAY									

CELIAC DISEASE COOKBOOK

Weekly Meal PLANNER

DATE ___ / ___ / ___

MONDAY

Breakfast |

Lunch |

Dinner |

Snack |

TUESDAY

Breakfast |

Lunch |

Dinner |

Snack |

WEDNESDAY

Breakfast |

Lunch |

Dinner |

Snack |

THURSDAY

Breakfast |

Lunch |

Dinner |

Snack |

FRIDAY

Breakfast |

Lunch |

Dinner |

Snack |

SATURDAY

Breakfast |

Lunch |

Dinner |

Snack |

SUNDAY

Breakfast |

Lunch |

Dinner |

Snack |

WATER INTAKE

Day									
MONDAY									
TUESDAY									
WEDNESDAY									
THURSDAY									
FRIDAY									
SATURDAY									
SUNDAY									

CELIAC DISEASE COOKBOOK

Weekly Meal PLANNER

DATE ___/___/___

MONDAY

Breakfast

Lunch

Dinner

Snack

TUESDAY

Breakfast

Lunch

Dinner

Snack

WEDNESDAY

Breakfast

Lunch

Dinner

Snack

THURSDAY

Breakfast

Lunch

Dinner

Snack

FRIDAY

Breakfast

Lunch

Dinner

Snack

SATURDAY

Breakfast

Lunch

Dinner

Snack

SUNDAY

Breakfast

Lunch

Dinner

Snack

WATER INTAKE

MONDAY	
TUESDAY	
WEDNESDAY	
THURSDAY	
FRIDAY	
SATURDAY	
SUNDAY	

CELIAC DISEASE COOKBOOK

Weekly Meal PLANNER

DATE ___/___/___

MONDAY

Breakfast |

Lunch |

Dinner |

Snack |

TUESDAY

Breakfast |

Lunch |

Dinner |

Snack |

WEDNESDAY

Breakfast |

Lunch |

Dinner |

Snack |

THURSDAY

Breakfast |

Lunch |

Dinner |

Snack |

FRIDAY

Breakfast |

Lunch |

Dinner |

Snack |

SATURDAY

Breakfast |

Lunch |

Dinner |

Snack |

SUNDAY

Breakfast |

Lunch |

Dinner |

Snack |

WATER INTAKE

| MONDAY |
| TUESDAY |
| WEDNESDAY |
| THURSDAY |
| FRIDAY |
| SATURDAY |
| SUNDAY |

CELIAC DISEASE COOKBOOK

Weekly Meal PLANNER

DATE ___ / ___ / ___

MONDAY

Breakfast

Lunch

Dinner

Snack

TUESDAY

Breakfast

Lunch

Dinner

Snack

WEDNESDAY

Breakfast

Lunch

Dinner

Snack

THURSDAY

Breakfast

Lunch

Dinner

Snack

FRIDAY

Breakfast

Lunch

Dinner

Snack

SATURDAY

Breakfast

Lunch

Dinner

Snack

SUNDAY

Breakfast

Lunch

Dinner

Snack

WATER INTAKE

| MONDAY |
| TUESDAY |
| WEDNESDAY |
| THURSDAY |
| FRIDAY |
| SATURDAY |
| SUNDAY |

CELIAC DISEASE COOKBOOK

Weekly Meal PLANNER

DATE ___/___/___

MONDAY

Breakfast |
Lunch |
Dinner |
Snack |

TUESDAY

Breakfast |
Lunch |
Dinner |
Snack |

WEDNESDAY

Breakfast |
Lunch |
Dinner |
Snack |

THURSDAY

Breakfast |
Lunch |
Dinner |
Snack |

FRIDAY

Breakfast |
Lunch |
Dinner |
Snack |

SATURDAY

Breakfast |
Lunch |
Dinner |
Snack |

SUNDAY

Breakfast |
Lunch |
Dinner |
Snack |

WATER INTAKE

| MONDAY |
| TUESDAY |
| WEDNESDAY |
| THURSDAY |
| FRIDAY |
| SATURDAY |
| SUNDAY |

CELIAC DISEASE COOKBOOK

Weekly Meal PLANNER

DATE ___ / ___ / ___

MONDAY

Breakfast |

Lunch |

Dinner |

Snack |

TUESDAY

Breakfast |

Lunch |

Dinner |

Snack |

WEDNESDAY

Breakfast |

Lunch |

Dinner |

Snack |

THURSDAY

Breakfast |

Lunch |

Dinner |

Snack |

FRIDAY

Breakfast |

Lunch |

Dinner |

Snack |

SATURDAY

Breakfast |

Lunch |

Dinner |

Snack |

SUNDAY

Breakfast |

Lunch |

Dinner |

Snack |

WATER INTAKE

MONDAY	
TUESDAY	
WEDNESDAY	
THURSDAY	
FRIDAY	
SATURDAY	
SUNDAY	

CELIAC DISEASE COOKBOOK

Weekly Meal PLANNER

DATE ___/___/___

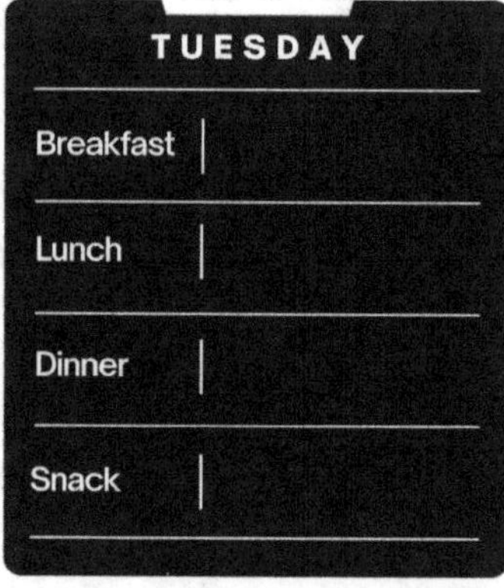

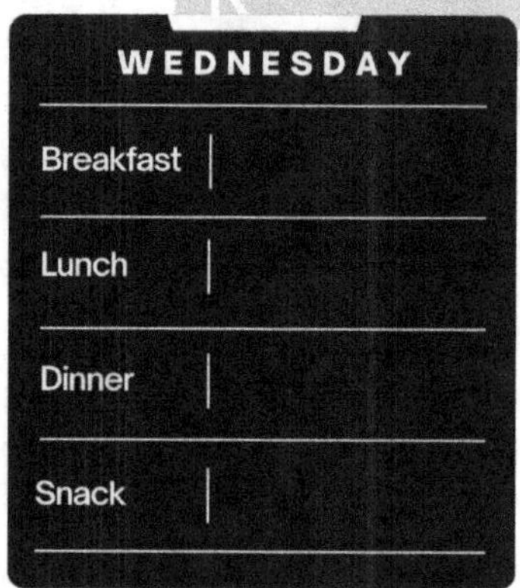

MONDAY

Breakfast |

Lunch |

Dinner |

Snack |

TUESDAY

Breakfast |

Lunch |

Dinner |

Snack |

WEDNESDAY

Breakfast |

Lunch |

Dinner |

Snack |

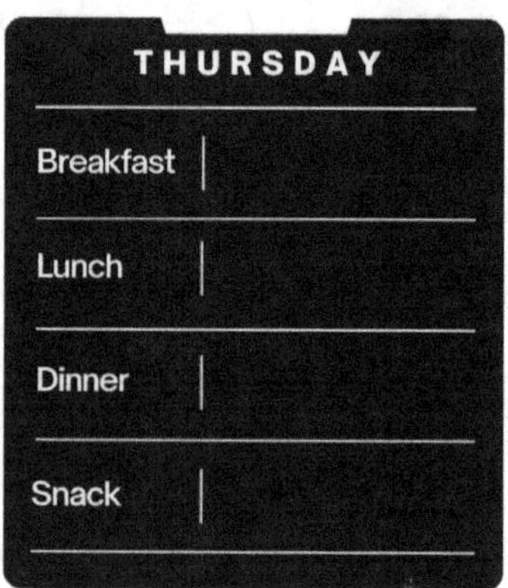

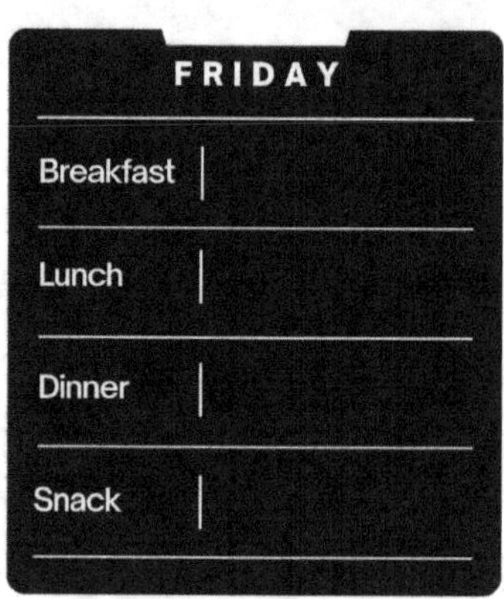

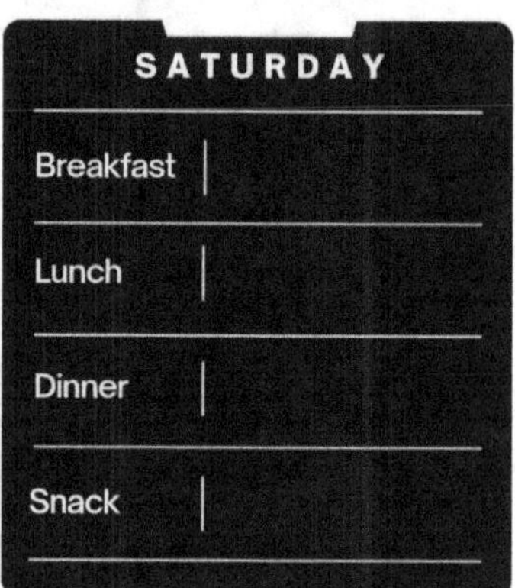

THURSDAY

Breakfast |

Lunch |

Dinner |

Snack |

FRIDAY

Breakfast |

Lunch |

Dinner |

Snack |

SATURDAY

Breakfast |

Lunch |

Dinner |

Snack |

SUNDAY

Breakfast |

Lunch |

Dinner |

Snack |

WATER INTAKE

MONDAY									
TUESDAY									
WEDNESDAY									
THURSDAY									
FRIDAY									
SATURDAY									
SUNDAY									

CELIAC DISEASE COOKBOOK

Weekly Meal PLANNER

DATE ___/___/___

MONDAY

Breakfast |

Lunch |

Dinner |

Snack |

TUESDAY

Breakfast |

Lunch |

Dinner |

Snack |

WEDNESDAY

Breakfast |

Lunch |

Dinner |

Snack |

THURSDAY

Breakfast |

Lunch |

Dinner |

Snack |

FRIDAY

Breakfast |

Lunch |

Dinner |

Snack |

SATURDAY

Breakfast |

Lunch |

Dinner |

Snack |

SUNDAY

Breakfast |

Lunch |

Dinner |

Snack |

WATER INTAKE

| MONDAY |
| TUESDAY |
| WEDNESDAY |
| THURSDAY |
| FRIDAY |
| SATURDAY |
| SUNDAY |

CELIAC DISEASE COOKBOOK

Weekly Meal PLANNER

DATE ___/___/___

MONDAY

Breakfast |

Lunch |

Dinner |

Snack |

TUESDAY

Breakfast |

Lunch |

Dinner |

Snack |

WEDNESDAY

Breakfast |

Lunch |

Dinner |

Snack |

THURSDAY

Breakfast |

Lunch |

Dinner |

Snack |

FRIDAY

Breakfast |

Lunch |

Dinner |

Snack |

SATURDAY

Breakfast |

Lunch |

Dinner |

Snack |

SUNDAY

Breakfast |

Lunch |

Dinner |

Snack |

WATER INTAKE									
MONDAY									
TUESDAY									
WEDNESDAY									
THURSDAY									
FRIDAY									
SATURDAY									
SUNDAY									

CELIAC DISEASE COOKBOOK

Weekly Meal PLANNER

DATE ___/___/___

MONDAY

Breakfast |

Lunch |

Dinner |

Snack |

TUESDAY

Breakfast |

Lunch |

Dinner |

Snack |

WEDNESDAY

Breakfast |

Lunch |

Dinner |

Snack |

THURSDAY

Breakfast |

Lunch |

Dinner |

Snack |

FRIDAY

Breakfast |

Lunch |

Dinner |

Snack |

SATURDAY

Breakfast |

Lunch |

Dinner |

Snack |

SUNDAY

Breakfast |

Lunch |

Dinner |

Snack |

WATER INTAKE

| MONDAY |
| TUESDAY |
| WEDNESDAY |
| THURSDAY |
| FRIDAY |
| SATURDAY |
| SUNDAY |

CELIAC DISEASE COOKBOOK

Weekly Meal PLANNER

DATE ___/___/___

MONDAY

Breakfast |

Lunch |

Dinner |

Snack |

TUESDAY

Breakfast |

Lunch |

Dinner |

Snack |

WEDNESDAY

Breakfast |

Lunch |

Dinner |

Snack |

THURSDAY

Breakfast |

Lunch |

Dinner |

Snack |

FRIDAY

Breakfast |

Lunch |

Dinner |

Snack |

SATURDAY

Breakfast |

Lunch |

Dinner |

Snack |

SUNDAY

Breakfast |

Lunch |

Dinner |

Snack |

WATER INTAKE

MONDAY								
TUESDAY								
WEDNESDAY								
THURSDAY								
FRIDAY								
SATURDAY								
SUNDAY								

CELIAC DISEASE COOKBOOK

Weekly Meal PLANNER

DATE ___/___/___

MONDAY

Breakfast |

Lunch |

Dinner |

Snack |

TUESDAY

Breakfast |

Lunch |

Dinner |

Snack |

WEDNESDAY

Breakfast |

Lunch |

Dinner |

Snack |

THURSDAY

Breakfast |

Lunch |

Dinner |

Snack |

FRIDAY

Breakfast |

Lunch |

Dinner |

Snack |

SATURDAY

Breakfast |

Lunch |

Dinner |

Snack |

SUNDAY

Breakfast |

Lunch |

Dinner |

Snack |

WATER INTAKE	
MONDAY	
TUESDAY	
WEDNESDAY	
THURSDAY	
FRIDAY	
SATURDAY	
SUNDAY	

CELIAC DISEASE COOKBOOK

Weekly Meal PLANNER

DATE ___/___/___

MONDAY

Breakfast |

Lunch |

Dinner |

Snack |

TUESDAY

Breakfast |

Lunch |

Dinner |

Snack |

WEDNESDAY

Breakfast |

Lunch |

Dinner |

Snack |

THURSDAY

Breakfast |

Lunch |

Dinner |

Snack |

FRIDAY

Breakfast |

Lunch |

Dinner |

Snack |

SATURDAY

Breakfast |

Lunch |

Dinner |

Snack |

SUNDAY

Breakfast |

Lunch |

Dinner |

Snack |

WATER INTAKE

MONDAY	
TUESDAY	
WEDNESDAY	
THURSDAY	
FRIDAY	
SATURDAY	
SUNDAY	

CELIAC DISEASE COOKBOOK

Weekly Meal PLANNER

DATE ___/___/___

MONDAY

Breakfast

Lunch

Dinner

Snack

TUESDAY

Breakfast

Lunch

Dinner

Snack

WEDNESDAY

Breakfast

Lunch

Dinner

Snack

THURSDAY

Breakfast

Lunch

Dinner

Snack

FRIDAY

Breakfast

Lunch

Dinner

Snack

SATURDAY

Breakfast

Lunch

Dinner

Snack

SUNDAY

Breakfast

Lunch

Dinner

Snack

WATER INTAKE

MONDAY	
TUESDAY	
WEDNESDAY	
THURSDAY	
FRIDAY	
SATURDAY	
SUNDAY	

CELIAC DISEASE COOKBOOK

Weekly Meal PLANNER

DATE ____ / ____ / ____

MONDAY
Breakfast |
Lunch |
Dinner |
Snack |

TUESDAY
Breakfast |
Lunch |
Dinner |
Snack |

WEDNESDAY
Breakfast |
Lunch |
Dinner |
Snack |

THURSDAY
Breakfast |
Lunch |
Dinner |
Snack |

FRIDAY
Breakfast |
Lunch |
Dinner |
Snack |

SATURDAY
Breakfast |
Lunch |
Dinner |
Snack |

SUNDAY
Breakfast |
Lunch |
Dinner |
Snack |

WATER INTAKE									
MONDAY									
TUESDAY									
WEDNESDAY									
THURSDAY									
FRIDAY									
SATURDAY									
SUNDAY									

CELIAC DISEASE COOKBOOK